Members

Steering Committee on Future Health Scenarios

J. van Londen, *chairman*
Director-General of Health
Ministry of Welfare, Health and Cultural Affairs, Rijswijk

Dr. J.L.A. Boelen
Director of Medical Affairs
St. Antonius Hospital
Nieuwegein

Dr. E. Borst-Eilers
Deputy chairwoman of the Health Council, The Hague

Dr. H.H. Cohen
Ex-Director-General of the National Institute for Health and Environmental Hygiene
Bilthoven

W.J.C. van Gestel, *M.D.*
Chief Medical Officer
Rijswijk

Dr. L. Ginjaar
Chairman of the Health Council
The Hague

Prof. dr. J.M. Greep
Faculty of Medicine
University of Limburg
Maastricht

Mr. J.P.M. Hendriks
Chairman of the National Council for Public Health
Zoetermeer

Dr. L.B.J. Stuyt
Ex-Chairman of the Health Council
The Hague

Prof. dr. H.M. Langeveld
Ex-member of the Netherlands Scientific Council of Government Policy, Professor of Emancipation Issues, University of Rotterdam

Dr. G.M. van Etten
Head of the Staff Bureau of Health Policy Development
Ministry of Welfare, Health and Cultural Affairs
Rijswijk

R.F. Schreuder, *LL.M. Secretary*
Ministry of Welfare, Health and Cultural Affairs
Rijswijk

Scenario Commission on Future Health Care Technology

Prof. dr. H.D. Banta, *Chairman*
c/o Health Council
The Hague

Prof. dr. D.W. van Bekkum
TNO Radiobiological Institute
Rijswijk

Prof. dr. J. Blanpain
Leuven University
Leuven
Belgium

Mrs. ir. M.H. Blom-Fuhri Snethlage
Netherlands Study Centre for Technology Trends
The Hague

Mrs. drs. S. Buitendijk
Yale University
School of Medicine
New Haven
U.S.A.

Prof. dr. H. Danielsson
Swedish Medical Research Council
Stockholm
Sweden

Prof. dr. H. Galjaard
Erasmus University
Rotterdam

Ir. C. Kramer
Philips Holland
Medical Systems/Plans and Programs
Eindhoven

Dr. P.W.J. Peters
National Institute of Health and Environmental Hygiene
Bilthoven

Prof. dr. D. de Wied
Rudolph Magnus Institute for Farmacology
Utrecht

Official Observers

Mrs. dr. E. Borst-Eilers
Deputy chairwoman of the Health Council
The Hague

Dr. L. Ginjaar
Chairman of the Health Council
The Hague

Prof. dr. J.M.L. Groot
State University of Limburg
Health Economics Group
Maastricht

Dr. J.W. Hartgerink
R.F. Schreuder, LL.M.
Ministry of Welfare, Health and Cultural Affairs
Staff Bureau of Health Policy Development
Rijswijk

Dr. H.G.M. Rigter
Executive Director of the Health Council
The Hague

Dr. J. Vang
World Health Organization (EURO)
Copenhagen
Denmark

Project Staff

Prof. dr. H.D. Banta
Project Director

Mrs. drs. A.C. Gelijns
Senior Researcher
(up to March 1987)

Drs. J. Griffioen
Researcher

Drs. P.J. Graaff
Researcher

Mrs. B. van der Lans
Secretary

Anticipating and Assessing Health Care Technology Volume 4

Scenario Commission on Future
Health Care Technology

chairman H. David Banta

senior researcher Annetine Gelijns

Anticipating and Assessing Health Care Technology Volume 4

Health Care Application of Lasers: The Future Treatment of Coronary Artery Disease

A report, commissioned by the
Steering Committee on Future Health Scenarios

1988
Kluwer Academic Publishers
Dordrecht – Boston – London

Distributors

for the United States and Canada: Kluwer Academic Publishers.
101 Philip Drive, Norwell, MA 02061, U.S.A.
For all other countries: Kluwer Academic Publishers Group,
P.O. Box 322, 3300 AH Dordrecht, The Netherlands

Steering Committee
on Future Health Scenarios
P.O. Box 5406
2280 HK Rijswijk
The Netherlands
Telephone: 070-407209

ISBN 978-94-011-6762-8 ISBN 978-94-011-6760-4 (eBook)
DOI 10.1007/978-94-011-6760-4

Foreword

This report, **Health Care Applications of Lasers: The Future Treatment of Coronary Artery Disease**, is the fourth report from the STG Commission on Future Health Care Technology and one of a series of case studies from that project. The STG (Stuurgroep Toekomstscenario's Gezondheidzorg) was established in 1983 as an independent advisory group to the State Secretary for Welfare, Public Health, and Cultural Affairs (WVC) to assist in long-range health planning efforts. Thus far, STG commissions have examined cardiovascular disease, cancer, aging, and life styles as issues of importance to the health of the Dutch population in the future.

Obviously, health care technology is of great concern to the government. On the one hand, technology is one of the major tools to promote a healthy population. On the other hand, the costs of health care have been rising at an alarming rate in recent years. These two facts, along with the social consequences of certain technologies such as genetic screening, led the STG to establish the Commission on Future Health Care Technology in 1985. The European Office of the World Health Organization (EURO) cosponsored the project. The Health Council (Gezondheidsraad) agreed to cooperate with the project by furnishing space and intellectual and logistical support.

The goal of the Commission's work is to develop sufficient information on future technological developments in health and health care to assist planning for their consequences.

The first report, **Anticipating and Assessing Health Care Technology**, gave the overall context for activities concerning future health care technology. The government and Dutch society as a whole must move rapidly to deal with the consequences of technological change in health care. The first report provided conclusions for achieving this purpose, focusing on the need to develop a national program or system of health care technology assessment.

The second report, **Future Technological Changes**, presented detailed information on anticipated future health care technologies. In the context of STG's studies, this might be considered an 'early warning system' for health care technology.

The third report, **Developments in the Regeneration, Repair and Reorganization of Nervous Tissue**, focused on future applications of neurosciences, especially regarding Alzheimer's disease, Parkinson's disease, and accidents involving nervous system trauma.

This report presents a general introduction to lasers in health care, although more detailed information is presented in Volume 2. The main purpose of this case study is to examine the possible impacts of one application of lasers: the treatment of coronary artery disease.

The fifth report, **Developments in Genetic Testing**, examines another application of the new biotechnology, the rapidly developing field of genetics. The genetic revolution has now truly begun and it will transform the ways that society deals with its genetic inheritance. The implications of this new technology are far-reaching. The report explores some of these implications and suggests the importance of careful monitoring of this field.

The sixth report, **Applications of the New Biotechnology: The Case of Vaccines**, discusses developments in the new biotechnology. The ability to directly manipulate the genetic structure of organisms has lead to dramatic changes in biological research, and is now beginning to transform practical technology as well. The report presents some of the new developments in diagnostic and therapeutic technologies. The main purpose of the report, however, is to point out the potential applications in vaccine development and possible future impacts of this field on the health of the Netherlands population.

The seventh report, **Computer Assisted Medical Imaging: The Case of Picture Archiving and Communications Systems (PACS)**, presents information on an important new technology. Since the early 1970s, departments of radiology have gradually turned to imaging with computers, and there are now predictions that all medical images, including conventional x-rays, will be computerized. Such a move would have great potential advantages, but the costs to the health care system and society would also be large. It is important for Dutch society to become aware of these developments and to determine the best course of future action.

The final report from the project on future health care technology, **Potentials for Home Care Technology**, gives an overview of present and future developments in an important and often-neglected field of health care. The report also describes and analyses the home care system of the Netherlands, and conlcudes that the home care system is not structured to be receptive to technology. Therefore, the report suggests ways that the home care system could be improved.

As Chairman of the STG, I am delighted to present this report, and I thank the Commission very sincerely for its rapid and excellent work. The government expects to see changes in policies toward health care technology, and I am certain that the report will be a substantial help in that process of change.

The report was prepared by the Commission's staff, which is listed in this report. The staff was led by Dr. David Banta, an American who agreed to spend two years with the STG chairing the Commission. The decision to invite Dr. Banta to the Netherlands was a recognition of the international nature of issues concerning health care technology. I would also like to point out the presence of a Swede, Dr. Henry Danielson, and a Belgian, Professor Jan Blanpain, on the Commission. Dr. Johannes Vang from WHO/EURO was an official observer on the Commission. We are particularly grateful to these outside guests.

The reports have been developed with the help of experts and reviewed by the Commission and by many other individuals and groups representing a wide range of disciplines and perspectives. We are grateful for their many contributions. As with all STG reports, however, the content of the report is the responsibility of the Commission and the STG and does not necessarily represent the position of any of those who assisted or of the Ministry of WVC.

J. van Londen
Chairman, STG

Preface

As noted in the Foreword, this report is one of several volumes resulting from this study of future health care technology.

The purpose of the study, as formulated by the STG, was to analyze future health care technology. Part of the task was to develop an 'early warning system' for health care technology. The primary goal of the project was to develop a list or description of a number of possible and probable future health care technologies, as well as information on their importance. Within the limits of time and money, this has been done. However, given the vast number of possible future health care technologies, complete information on the importance of each area could not be developed in any depth for all technology.

Therefore, four specific technologies were chosen and were prospectively assessed. These future technologies were examined in more depth, looking particularly at their future health and policy implications. Subsequently, the project was extended to September 1986, and two additional technologies will be assessed.

The total output of the project is as follows:

Volume 1. GENERAL CONSIDERATIONS AND POLICY RECOMMENDATIONS

Volume 2. FUTURE TECHNOLOGICAL CHANGES

Volume 3. DEVELOPMENTS IN THE REGENERATION, REPAIR AND REORGANIZATION OF NERVOUS TISSUE

Volume 4. HEALTH CARE APPLICATIONS OF LASERS: THE FUTURE TREATMENT OF CORONARY ARTERY DISEASE

Volume 5. DEVELOPMENTS IN GENETIC TESTING

Volume 6. APPLICATIONS OF THE NEW BIOTECHNOLOGY: The Case of Vaccines

Volume 7. COMPUTER-ASSISTED MEDICAL IMAGING: The Case of Picture Archiving and Communications Systems (PACS)

Volume 8. POTENTIALS FOR HOME CARE TECHNOLOGY

The first report was addressed to an important purpose. The Commission reached the tentative conclusion early in its deliberations that a system for identifying future health care technology would be of limited benefit on its own. The Netherlands does not have an organized system for technology assessment in health care, and therefore information on the benefits, risks, financial costs, and social implications of technology is not available for new or established technology, generally speaking. The Commission saw the need for such a system. Studies aimed at the identification and assessment of future health care technologies must be developed within such a context, the Commission concluded. Therefore, Volume I was developed as an overall policy document, and contains summary material on future technologies. This report gives the detailed information on the same technologies and technological areas.

The second report presented overall information on future health care technology. The report was based on information obtained from surveys done in the United States and in Europe.

The case studies are intended to examine important areas of future (and emerging) health care technology. However, many other potential subjects and applications could be examined. This case study, then, is only an example of what may be possible in evaluating the impacts of future health care technology.

Technological developments in health care are occurring rapidly, and the information on future technologies in these report will rapidly become out-of-date. The Commission is aware of this fact, and hopes that it will be possible to continue an 'early warning system' that will periodically update such information and assess specific technologies.

This report is primarily addressed to policy makers and to those who are interested in national level policy making. At the same time, the Commission believes that the information in this report is an important basis for future activities in health care technology assessment in Netherlands and in other countries.

Dr. H. David Banta
Chairman
Commission on Future Health Care Technology

Table of Contents

List of Tables

List of Figures

Introduction

The term 'laser' is the acronym for **L**ight **A**mplification by **S**timulated **E**mission of **R**adiation. Laser technology produces a highly focused, high power source of energy. One of its most important effects is that it can be converted to heat at a specific target point. The principle of the laser was described by Einstein in 1917, when he predicted that an excited atom capable of emitting a photon of a certain frequency would be stimulated to do so by radiation of that frequency, and that the likelihood of stimulated emission would be proportional to the intensity of the stimulating radiation (44). Einstein also inferred that the radiation emitted would be highly directional. Other characteristics of the light emitted include that it is monochromatic (of one color). (Technical aspects of lasers are further discussed in Appendix A of this report.)

Functional lasers became available about 25 years ago. They have found rapid application in many areas, even including reading compact discs in many homes (52). This case concerns applications in health care, focusing on potential future applications in treatment of coronary artery atherosclerotic disease.

General applications of lasers in health care were reviewed in Volume II, **Future Technological Changes**, from this project. This material, therefore, will be only briefly summarized in this report.

Section 1 – Lasers in Health Care

Background

After their development, lasers were rapidly applied to a variety of scientific ends in physics, meteorology, astronomy, medicine, and industry (36). Chemists quickly saw the value of devices that could stimulate molecules in specific ways and in short periods of time, compared with techniques available at the time. Specific knowledge of the role of chlorophyll in photosynthesis was one result (44). By now, the influence of lasers is pervasive in most scientific fields. They are used to monitor geological structures, to measure the constituents of the upper atmosphere, and to study the dynamics of the Solar System (44).

Lasers have increasingly found practical applications. Lasers are now used in communications, industry, defense, and medicine. In communications, information is transmitted via laser light traveling in small optical fibers. In industry, lasers are used for many purposes, including drilling, cutting, welding, and surface treatment. In defense, laser radar and laser target designators are already in use, and laser weapons seem likely in the future. And in medicine, lasers are already used in both treatment (especially in surgery) and diagnosis (52). The main subject of this report is medical applications, focusing on the now-experimental use of lasers in treating coronary artery disease.

The three lasers common in health care are the carbon dioxide (CO_2) laser, the argon laser, and the Nd-YAG laser (9). In one medical center in 1983, 55 percent of procedures used argon, 30 percent CO_2, and 15 percent Nd-YAG. In 8 percent, more than one wavelength was used (19). However, with the growing use of carbon dioxide and Nd-YAG lasers in surgery, these figures are probably no longer realistic (the argon laser is used primarily in ophthalmology). New types of lasers, such as dye lasers, excimer lasers, and semi-conductor lasers, are beginning to find applications in health care (8;9;53).

Laser technology has changed rapidly. The original CO_2 laser sources were very large and bulky. CO_2 lasers are now small and portable. Likewise, Argon lasers are now much smaller. Nd-YAG lasers are still large and heavy due to their associated water cooling system (19). The technology is not changing very rapidly now, but the delivery system for the laser beam is evolving, so that less power is needed than was true in the past (9).

A laser beam from a CO_2 laser does not pass through a fiber well, so it cannot be used as a part of an endoscope system. Fibers do conduct argon laser energy reasonably well. Nd-YAG laser beams can also be conducted by fibers. Technological improvements in use of lasers with endoscopes can be expected (19). Fuller (23) has reviewed fiberoptics and endoscopy with lasers.

Use of lasers in surgical cutting in general is done by direct application of the laser beam from the end of a quartz fiber. This has led to problems in cardiovascular surgery, such as perforation of a blood vessel (17). A recent development uses so- called 'tips' made of either metal or sapphire mounted at the end of the quartz fiber (1). The metal tip is a metal cap mounted at the distal end of the laser fiber. The laser acts as a heat source. Even more recently, sapphire tips have been mounted at the end of the laser fiber for surgical use (6;21). These tips, which are available in various shapes, become hot, but they also emit laser light.

Research Applications

Lasers have a number of applications in basic research. For example, they are used in high resolution spectroscopy. The behavior of laser light can be used to make highly sensitive instruments. Even a single atom or molecule can be detected (40). As computers are linked with lasers more and more, more applications are certain. Health-related research is linked to instruments also used in diagnosis, described below.

Applications in Diagnosis

Diagnostic applications of lasers have their roots in chemistry and physics. Low-intensity laser light is absorbed, reflected, or reradiated by the substance causing minimal changes within it. This is the basis for diagnostic applications, both at the atomic and molecular level and at the macroscopic level (such as motion and shape of cells and organs). In addition, lasers can be used to excite biologically important molecules for research and diagnostic purposes (41).

The diagnostic applications of lasers are still largely in development, but some of the applications described below seem certain to spread into routine use with time.

Laser radiation can be used to measure the position, velocity, shape, and so forth of various components of biological objects. One of the first biomedical applications was in flow cytometry, where the laser was used in the rapid analysis and separation of individual cells by accurately measuring their optical properties (particularly by laser-induced fluorescence) (41). Great progress has been made in clinical immunology through the use of laser cytofluorometry. Flow cytofluorometry is used to identify ribonucleic acid (RNA) and deoxyribonucleic acid (DNA) in blood plasma and abnormal cells in Pap smears, as well as to separate white cells from blood and to study cellular kinetics in leukemia. Flow cytofluorometry has also been used to identify different cell nuclei in hybrid cell populations and in the isolation of individual human chromosomes. Both approaches have contributed to the mapping of normal and mutant human genes.

Another interesting area of development is to use laser holographic techniques to produce three-dimensional medical images (41). The contours of biological objects can be mapped and their deformations analyzed. Such instruments are being considered for use in such fields as orthopedics, radiology, ophthalmology, neurosurgery, urology, otology, and dentistry.

An x-ray laser is in development (37), which has research consequences, but may also lead to new forms of medical imaging.

Applications in Therapy

The major therapeutic application of lasers now is in surgery, although other applications may become more prominent in the future (9). Procedures traditionally done by surgeons are now being replaced by procedures done by other specialists, such as cardiologists and radiologists. Technically speaking, these are not 'surgical' procedures, although some of the medical literature describes them as such. In this report, only use of a laser in a procedure by a surgical specialist is considered as surgery.

Surgery. The laser has advantages as a surgical tool because it can vaporize and remove tissue without touching it. Because the laser cauterizes (closes by burning) blood vessels, there is reduced blood loss and a clear operative field. Lasers may be considered fully established in some areas of surgery, such as ophthalmology and dermatology (4;19;32;33;39). In ophthalmology, use of the argon laser in retinal detachment and of the Nd-YAG laser in cataract extraction are fully accepted (4;48;49), with such experimental applications as excimer lasers in corneal surgery. In dermatologic surgery, the laser is fully accepted in the removal of such skin lesions as tattoos and birthmarks (9;19;49).

The use of lasers in surgery has been adequately evaluated in only a few of the newer areas of surgical application. The carbon dioxide laser is generally used, and has the advantage of giving an accurate depth of incision. It also has the advantages of less bleeding; sealing of lymphatic vessels; no or less postoperative edema; and minimal spread of malignancy (cancer) during surgery (19;54). Lasers are now being used in tumor surgery (55); urological surgery (19); head and neck surgery (31); breast surgery (19); neurosurgery (5); ear, nose, and throat surgery (19); gynecological surgery for such problems as focal cancer of the cervix (57); and plastic surgery (19). Many procedures that previously were done in hospital can now be done in the office with lasers, particularly in gynecological surgery.

Other possible applications of lasers in specific areas of surgery are reviewed by Dixon (19). An area of particular interest is using lasers in treating cardiovascular disease instead of surgery. This subject is reviewed below.

The advantages of lasers over conventional surgical techniques make them likely to be widely used in the future in many types of surgery.

Treatment of Cardiovascular Disease. The basic task in treating cardiovascular disease with lasers is to remove a blockage, such as an atherosclerotic plaque (or atheroma), either partially or completely. Lasers are used thermally (12;13). They are passed to the site of the obstruction in a catheter and then heat the material blocking the vessel to such a temperature that it is vaporized, producing a new vessel lumen. For this approach to be successful, two different and independent types of problems must be solved: preventing damage to the vessel wall and finding the optimal method of delivering heat and light to the site of the obstruction (25;26).

Although early expectations were for use of lasers in the coronary arteries, useful clinical applications at this time are largely confined to the peripheral arteries (2;11;14;30;45). The procedure is usually done by cardiologists or radiologists.

Peripheral vascular surgery is often necessary to remove plaque and thrombi (clots) from vessels or to bypass areas of blockage in blood vessels. Some type of procedure to treat this condition is done about 6,000 times a year in the Netherlands (60). If the lesion in the blood vessel is localized, it is usual to do angioplasty by the Dotter procedure unless the vessel is completely blocked. A balloon-tipped catheter is passed through the artery to the site of the narrowing and inflation of the balloon reduces the obstruction. It can only be done in the larger arteries of the upper leg. This procedure was done 1,077 times in the Netherlands in 1984 (60). More extensive lesions are treated by a bypass operation using the sapphenous vein as the first choice of graft material. In 1984, 5,115 such procedures were done in the Netherlands (60). Recurrences occur in about 25 percent and are treated with autologous (artificial) grafts (16;20). Results with artificial grafts are not as good as those with sapphenous veins. Ultimately, amputation may be necessary when the blood vessels distal to the blockage are too diseased for the situation to be helped by bypass. Amputation was done in 2,307 cases in the Netherlands in 1984 (60).

In the early 1980's, it was shown that laser energy from argon, Nd-YAG or CO_2 lasers was able to ablate human (cadaver) atherosclerotic plaques to create a new lumen. Successful in vivo animal experiences were reported in 1982 (11). In 1984, the first clinical recanalization of a femoral artery was reported by Ginsburg (29), using an argon laser. Geschwind et al (27) used the Nd-YAG laser for recanalization of human femoral arteries. In England, Cumberland et al (14;15) revascularized human femoral and coronary arteries.

Using a bare fiber to recanalize blood vessels causes a relatively high incidence of immediate perforations (7). Unacceptable rates of recurrence are also thought to be a problem. Such early problems may be solved through the use of tips, mentioned earlier. Cumberland, Sanborn, and coworkers (14), for example, use the device to recanalize occluded peripheral arteries by moving the probe back and forth. About 10 watts of argon laser power is used. Clinical results are very promising so far. Large occlusions, up to 35 cm, can be recanalized with a lumen of about 1 mm. Balloon dilatation (PTCA) is part of the procedure. Immediate perforation of the vessel wall is substantially reduced. The danger of wall damage due to heat conduction from the hot tip is minimized by moving the probe continuously. About 150 patients all over the world have now been treated in this way. The first percutaneous laser-assisted coronary angioplasty in the human was reported by Cumberland et al in June 1986 (15), using a similar technique. The metal tip was used to create a channel in the obstructed coronary artery large enough to allow a dilatation balloon catheter through the site of the obstruction. Sapphire tips may have applications in the cardiovascular area. Their characteristics are something like bare fiber and something like the metal heater cap. If the advantages of the two systems can be combined, minimizing disadvantages, these tips may become useful. Sapphire tips have already been used to recanalize obstructed arteries in amputated limbs (6) and in a few patients (21). Tips, which have only been used recently, seem to be a breakthrough in clinical use of lasers in cardiovascular treatment.

Another problem with laser angioplasty is the tendency for the vessel to be closed again by formation of a clot or thrombus at the site of the previous lesion.

Recent work has focused on the possibilities of ultraviolet pulsed excimer lasers (8;17;33;34;46). They have been used in vitro and have been successful. They have not been used in vivo because it is difficult to couple the light into a fiber without shattering the proximal end of the fiber tip.

Another type of cardiovascular disease, cardiac arrhythmias, may also be treated in the future with lasers. In arrhythmias, an electrical focus in the heart causes an irregularity of heart rhythm. This focus could be removed using a laser in a catheter in many cases. This may become the accepted treatment in the future.

Treatment of coronary artery disease will be reviewed in Section 3.

Other Possible Future Medical Treatments Involving Lasers. Nd-YAG lasers are being used in conjunction with endoscopes to seal bleeding blood vessels, for example in the stomach (38). Early reports indicate that treating a bleeding peptic ulcer in this way reduced the rebleeding rate and the need for emergency surgery. For example, of 70 patients with bleeding peptic ulcer, 7 bled again after laser therapy, while of 68 patients treated conventionally, 27 bled again (62). Several randomized trials are underway of this technique, and a detailed cost analysis is being done in England.

Lasers can fragment stones in the ureter when passed up the ureter with an endoscope. Watson and Wickham (63) have used a pulsed dye laser to fragment such stones with minimal or no damage to ureteric tissue. By November 1986, 75 cases had been treated in this way. While still experimental, this procedure has promise for the future.

Photobiology and photomedicine. These therapeutic applications depend on the laser's ability to photo-excite biological molecules (24). Applications so far have been based on the fact that acted upon by low-intensity light a molecule can absorb no more than one photon (41). One-photon phototherapy has been used in treating neonatal jaundice, various skin diseases such as psoriasis, and cancer. The use of phototherapy in cancer is still experimental, however. Since laser radiation can be delivered to internal organs through an endoscope, phototherapy could also be used with endoscopes.

In the future, photodynamic (or photosensitization) therapy could spread rapidly. This therapy utilizes the photosensitizing and tumor localizing properties of certain substances, especially porphyrins, in the treatment of malignancies (19). A photosensitizer is administered intravenously in this technique and spreads throughout the body. For reasons not understood, the substance is retained in premalignant and malignant tissue for a longer time than in normal tissue. Laser energy initiates a photodynamic process, resulting in tumor necrosis (death of cells). Present work includes trials for cancer of the eye, cancer of the bladder (58), and glioblastoma, a brain tumor (56). Clinical trials are needed to define the exact place of photodynamic therapy in cancer treatment (59).

Work is now also proceeding on two-photon excitation, which causes a more intense radiation. This may make phototherapy more effective in the future (41). However, two-photon radiation may also be more likely to be carcinogenic.

Soft Lasers. The field of 'soft lasers' is rapidly growing. These are weak helium-neon or infrared diode lasers using low power (up to tens of milliwatts). Lasers are now being used as an adjunct in acupuncture, for direct pain relief (as after surgery for wisdom tooth removal), for physiotherapy, and even in beauty salons for wrinkle removal. Physiotherapists use them for arthritis, hematomas (traumatic collections of blood), and sport accidents. Lasers are even used for this purpose on race horses. Clinical use of these soft lasers has preceded the proof of existence of a biostimulation phenomenon, although studies to investigate possible effects are being conducted now. If the phenomenon exists at all, there is no good idea as to what its mechanism of action is.

Safety of Lasers

The powerful light beams generated by lasers can be transmitted for some distance, are sometimes invisible, and can produce unique tissue reactions. These attributes are associated with specific safety problems. The greatest concern is the eyes of the patient and of personnel using the laser device. Special goggles or glasses must be worn while a laser is being used. Some feel that doors of rooms where a laser is being operated should be equipped with a switch to shut off the laser if the door is suddenly opened. However, others point out that this can cause danger to the patient, for example during treatment of a bleeding ulcer, when the laser would be shut off because someone entered the room.

Instruments used in a laser field must have a rough surface, so that a diffuse reflection will result in case of contact with the laser beam.

Any material used with the laser must not be flammable, since fire is always a potential hazard. In endoscopic surgery, fire is a particular hazard, especially with anesthesia. Endoscopes have caught fire in the past, especially in procedures involving the trachea and bronchi (tubes in the lungs). Various corporations are working on tubes that would be less flammable. High concentrations of oxygen are dangerous with lasers. On the other hand, several surgical procedures can be done through endoscopes without anesthesia except when an area close to a body orifice is involved. This has allowed more frequent ambulatory treatment of such conditions as bladder cancer, which makes the procedure safer (19).

Laser devices must generally meet performance standards which help to assure safety. In addition, high electrical power is needed, so adequate electrical lines are necessary. More electrical injuries than optical injuries have occurred in industry (19).

At the institutional level, it is important to control and monitor laser use. Dixon (19) has stressed the importance of a laser safety officer to monitor laser use to ensure safety for patients and operating room personnel. Access to a laser needs to be controlled as well, so that only those who have demonstrated proficiency with lasers are allowed to use them.

Cost Implications of Laser Equipment

The market for lasers is an active one, growing about 30 percent a year. In 1984, total sales of equipment in the United States were about US$200 million, according to one source, with projected sales of US$268 million in 1985 (40). In 1984 and 1985, specific figures for sales were as follows: Nd-YAG, $70 million in 1984, $95 million in 1985; argon-ion, $60 million in 1984, $78 million in 1985; CO2, $55 million in 1984, $77 million in 1985. Other types have much lower sales figures. Sales are projected to reach $800 million in the United States by 1990.

Another source gives even more optimistic figures (35). A market survey estimated that 1984 sales were US364 million, and projected 1985 sales of $465 million. The most rapidly growing market in the United States at the moment is sales of Nd-YAG lasers for posterior capsulotomy post-cataract (a form of eye surgery). During 1985 and 1986, 3000 systems were expected to be sold at an average price of US$80,000 (35).

In the near future, the most active market for lasers is expected to be among gastrointestinal physicians and urologists (see discussion of health care applications of lasers, above), with an annual potential number of procedures of 2 million in the United States (35). In the future, manufacturers expect laser angioplasty (procedures involving the blood vessels) to grow rapidly. In addition, manufacturers expect CO_2 lasers to continue to find new surgical applications and to grow in sales by 30 to 40 percent per year.

Fully equipped carbon dioxide lasers cost from US$25,000 to US$106,000. Argon lasers cost from US$25,000 to US$65,000. Nd-YAG lasers cost from $80,000 to $106,000 (19). The prices, however, are gradually coming down.

The period of obsolescence for a laser device is probably 3-5 years. Instrumentation is changing rapidly. Laser equipment is still bulky and subject to considerable down time (19), although newer instruments have improved reliability.

The costs do not include the costs of associated equipment, such as microscopes. In addition, special facilities are necessary, especially provisions for a special electrical power supply and water cooling to carry away excess heat. Technological improvements can also be expected here. The argon laser needs a new tube every 3-5 years at a cost of approximately US$10,000. The metal tips costs about US$450 each at the moment, but the price will come down. It is also possible that they may be re-used.

It is important to realize that the capital cost of the laser equipment may be a relatively small part of the overall cost of operating a laser. If a laser life is at least five years, it is standard practice to depreciate its value over that time. Other costs associated with a laser include maintenance and spare parts, interest on the loan, remodeling, technical staff, and supplies (such as tubes). Table 1 presents an estimate of the annual expense of operating a CO_2 laser in an operating theatre.

The cost of any one application would then depend on the calculated number of times the instrument is used. This figure can be estimated initially, based on manufacturer's recommendations and expected intensity of use. If the laser were used once a day, and the expense was maximal (that is, US$86,000 for a year), the cost per use would be more than US$400. If the laser were used four times a day, and the expense were minimal (that is, US$34,000), the expense per use would be approximately US$40. The overall cost of equipping and using an operating theatre is not available, but this is probably a small part of such an overall cost.

The assumption here is that the laser would be used in the operating room with this incremental cost. There would be no additional space or professional cost.

The cost-effectiveness of the use of lasers needs to be considered for any application. Strictly speaking, all costs and all benefits should be calculated. Using a cost-effectiveness technique would allow an outcome measure such as quality-adjusted life years (OTA, 1981), which would include 'softer' issues such as pain and functioning as well as mortality. The laser may improve certain procedures or make new procedures possible. Cost-effectiveness analysis can help indicate if the investment in these procedures is worthwhile.

At the same time, it is likely that in many cases the issue for lasers will be whether the overall cost of providing the procedure has increased. The first question to ask is whether the laser is as effective as the previous procedure (a surgical procedure, for example). If the effectiveness is roughly the same, then it is necessary to find out what the overall cost difference is. This will require special analysis. Some examples of effects of lasers that could be cost-lowering include:

1. the treatment of gastrointestinal bleeding by lasers could shorten length of stay in the hospital and cut down on the cost of other types of care. A study of this type is underway in England. However, it has the problem that costs only on the one hospitalization are being considered, whereas overall costs might include the necessity for rehospitalization;
2. use of a laser in surgery may be associated with lower rates of infection and serious bleeding, which could save medical costs;
3. surgery (for example, removal of a tumor in the gastrointestinal tract) done through an endoscope would generally be associated with a shorter length of stay in hospital and fewer complications. However, such factors as recurrence of disease and rehospitalization would then need to be considered;
4. laser treatment (including surgery) could perhaps be done more often without hospitalization, saving the expense of hospital beds.

Overall, lasers offer the prospect of decreasing the need for surgeons, operating rooms, and in-patient (or intramural) care. With lasers, other specialists may do procedures previously done by surgeons. Surgery may be done outside of the hospital. However, to realize economies the numbers of surgeons, operating theatres, and hospital beds would have to fall.

Specific calculations projecting possible future costs of lasers in coronary artery procedures are presented later in the report.

Section 2 – The Present Use of Lasers in Health Care in the Netherlands

The present use of lasers in health care in the Netherlands is somewhat limited. There is no clinical laser center where several lasers (such as CO_2, Nd-YAG, Argon, and Argon pumped dye) are in clinical use for the various medical specialties. There is also no research institute dealing with laser applications.

Lasers are largely confined clinically to ophthalmology and endoscopy. Lasers are now universal in eye surgery. Use of Nd-YAG lasers in endoscopy, especially in palliation of cancer, is growing rapidly in the Netherlands.

The laser expertise that exists is scattered over the country in both academic and larger non-university hospitals. Some of the more important centers include:

- Photodynamic therapy is done mainly in Rotterdam
- Oral surgery with lasers in Groningen
- ENT surgery with lasers in Groningen
- Urologic surgery in Amsterdam (AvL)
- Gastrointestinal applications in Amsterdam (AMC) and other hospitals
- Dermatological applications in Eindhoven
- Experimental cardiovascular work in Utrecht, Delft, and Eindhoven

Lasers have not been applied to neurosurgery or orthopedic surgery in the Netherlands. New laser applications, such as fragmentation of ureter stones, tissue welding, and excimer laser ablation (e.g., corneal surgery) are not being studied or developed in the Netherlands. In this respect, the Netherlands is at least five years behind such countries as France, England, Germany, and the United States.

Section 3 – Lasers in the Future Treatment of Coronary Artery Disease

Cardiovascular disease is one of the most prevalent diseases in industrialized societies, and one type of cardiovascular disease, ischemic heart disease, is highly significant. In the Netherlands, ischemic heart disease (when the heart does not receive enough blood in relation to demand due to blood vessel blockage from coronary artery disease) accounted for 14,948 deaths in men and 9,657 deaths in women in 1983, 21 percent of all deaths that year (60). Ischemic heart disease is the leading cause of death in men over the age of 35 and in all persons after the age of 50 (61). Symptoms from such heart disease are common, but even more people have serious disease without clinical symptoms.

Ischemic cardiovascular disease results from the process of atherosclerosis. Plaques are laid down in the arteries and cause a lack of oxygen to tissues served by those arteries. The result can be pain (angina pectoris in the case of the heart), acute necrosis (death) of tissues, as in acute myocardial infarction, chronic problems such as gangrene of the limbs, and even death.

Below, the present treatment of coronary artery disease is described. The important issue concerns the future place of laser treatment. If it works, the benefit in both health and financial terms could be substantial. This is indicated in the scenarios that are presented later in the report.

Present Treatment of Coronary Artery Disease

When coronary artery disease is recognized, its treatment depends on its severity and symptoms. Such conservative measures as altering diet, undertaking consistent exercize, and ceasing the smoking of cigarettes can be of value.

However, coronary artery disease generally comes to attention of a health care provider because of symptoms. With severe coronary artery obstruction, the heart muscle receives an inadequate supply of blood and oxygen, and the patient experiences chest pain (angina pectoris) either during exercize, with strong emotions, or in cold weather. With near-total obstruction, the pain may occur at rest or with minimal exertion. When angina pectoris is recognized, it is a sign of relatively far-advanced coronary artery disease. At this point, medical (as opposed to surgical) management of the problem is generally undertaken. Aside from prudent measures such as changing diet, drugs are helpful. Commonly used drugs are nitrates, beta blockers, and calcium antagonists. These drugs reduce the oxygen requirements of the heart, but do not affect the problem of lack of blood and oxygen.

Heart failure can also occur in coronary artery disease, with or without angina. Heart failure is treated with such drugs as digitalis to improve the contractions of the heart and diuretics to remove excess fluid from the body. Salt restriction may also be helpful.

All of the drugs may be used in various combinations. Treatment of coronary artery disease medically can thus be very complicated.

A serious consequence of coronary artery disease is myocardial infarction, or 'heart attack'. The infarction, irreversible death of cardiac tissue, occurs because of lack of oxygen to the cells caused by abrupt thrombosis (closing) in the remaining lumen of a narrowed coronary artery. The same drugs can be used during the acute period. In addition, thrombolytic therapy, the use of pharmacologic agents to lyse (dissolve) coronary thrombi (clots) early after an infarct, is being investigated. After recovery from a myocardial infarction, symptoms such as angina pectoris are common. However, angina may also disappear because the damaged tissue causing the pain previously has died.

If medical therapy of coronary artery disease fails (symptoms of severe chest pain are not relieved by therapy), restoration of the blood flow to the heart muscle must be considered. As with peripheral arterial disease, blockages must be removed or bypassed when they occur in the coronary arteries. A surgical procedure is coronary artery bypass graft (CABG). Angioplasty by a catheter balloon is another alternative. The intervention chosen depends on the extent of the coronary artery narrowing. If it is multiple, surgery is usually done. If it consists of a single lesion within reach of a catheter, balloon dilatation is usually the choice. If the thrombus is identified when an infarction is beginning, enzyme administration is often used. These alternatives, including lysing the clots, are not mutually exclusive.

Bypass operations involve introducing a graft of the sapphenous vein to connect the aorta to points distal to the obstruction(s). Coronary artery bypass was done almost 4,000 times in the Netherlands in 1981. The Health Council expects the need for bypass procedures to be 8,250 in 1990 (28). The STG scenarios (61) agree generally with this figure, but show sharp drop-offs after 1990, as the waiting lists for the procedure are ended and the age-adjusted death rates from ischemic heart disease continue to decline (see Figures 1 and 2). The fall in age-adjusted death rates reflects a fall in the underlying age-specific death rates. Because of the sharp increase in age-specific death rates from ischemic heart disease with age, a decline in these age-specific rates, as shown in Figure 2, indicates a delay in the onset of the disease of 5 to 7 years for both men and women. The decrease in absolute incidence, number of new cases per year, and prevalence of the disease (number of cases present) is only about 10 percent. Because of competing causes of death at older ages, the gain in life-expectancy from this change is also much smaller than 5 to 7 years, only about 2 months.

Candidates for bypass are identified by a variety of means. Severe angina pectoris not adequately relieved by drug treatment is the chief reason to consider surgery. The patient's electrocardiogram and exercize tolerance test would often be abnormal. Cardiac radionuclide imaging and echocardiography can be abnormal also. However, the operability of coronary artery disease can only be evaluated by coronary angiography to evaluate the obstruction. This is done by cardiac catheterization, which requires 15 minutes to 1 hour and involves introduction of catheters through arteries in either the arm or leg. Dye that can be seen on an x-ray (radioopaque) is injected into the coronary arteries and the blockages visualized by x-ray. Ventriculography and hemodynamic measurements are also done to assess the function of the left ventricle of the heart.

Coronary disease is life-threatening and surgery is frequently done in an emergency situation, when the patient has progressive angina pectoris or other signs of a threatening myocardial infarction. A coronary bypass operation, involving physically opening the chest, has a relatively high mortality in such circumstances. This indicates that lasers might be quite valuable in the future in this setting, since the procedure is less traumatic for the patient.

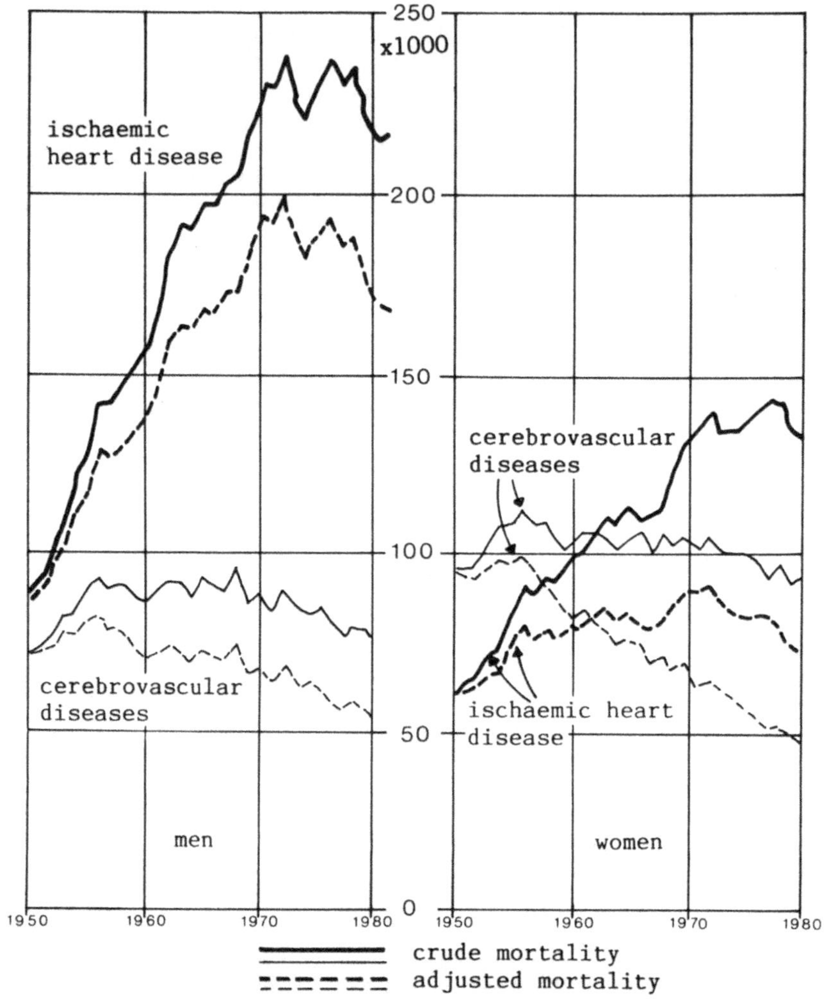

ischaemic heart disease:
1950-1968: I.C.D. 1948 and 1955 #420-422.1
1969-1980: I.C.D. 1965 and 1975 #410-414

cerebrovascular diseases:
1950-1968: I.C.D. 1948 and 1955 #330-334
1969-1980: I.C.D. 1965 and 1975 #430-438

Figure 1 Mortality due to IHD since 1950 in the Netherlands, for men and women, crude and age-adjusted rates
Standard population: 1950

Source: CBS, 1983, p. 152.

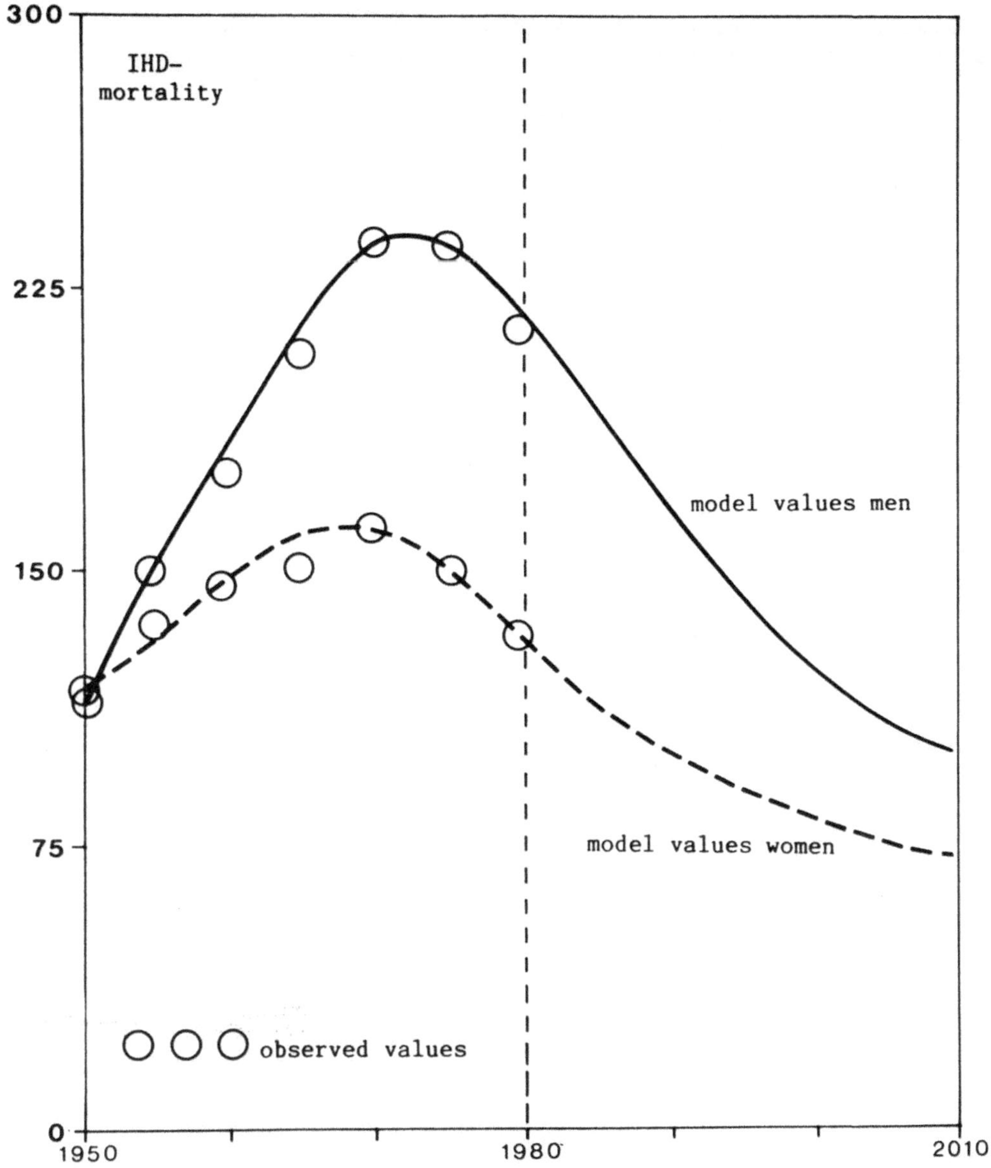

Figure 2 Adjusted IHD-mortalities, per 100,000, as observed and as calculated with the model, for Dutch men and women Standard population as in 1980

Source: 61

One significant problem with existing techniques is the lack of appropriate veins, especially if the saphenous vein has already been used. Another is difficulties in carrying out a second operative procedure in a person already operated because of fibrosis from the previous operation, especially with diffuse sclerosis.

A partial substitute for CABG is percutaneous transluminal angioplasty (PTCA). This technique involves passage of a balloon tipped catheter to the site of the arterial narrowing and inflation of the balloon to reduce the obstruction. The balloon apparently compresses the atherosclerotic plaque and stretches the arterial wall. When the person has short, segmental, and high grade (more than 50 percent) blockage of the coronary artery, he or she is a particularly good candidate for this alternative. Immediate success rates of the procedure range from 40 to 90 percent, depending on the characteristics of the disease and the skill of the clinician. Restenosis (closing of the artery) occurs in 25 to 35 percent of patients, usually within 6 months of the procedure (3).

Prospects for Laser Treatment of Coronary Artery Disease

Many workers have recanalized coronary arteries with lasers in cadavers and in animals (10;34). Choy et al (11) performed the first intra-operative coronary artery recanalizations in living human patients, using an Argon laser coupled to a bare fiber. Others have used a laser in a similar way during heart surgery (41;42). Crea et al (13) reported the first intra-operative use of the metal tip. Cumberland et al (16) reported its first percutaneous use (by catheter through the blood vessels of the leg) in humans.

Possibilities with lasers in cardiovascular surgery include (25;34): 1) to delay vascular surgery to preserve the saphenous vein as long as possible; 2) to be able to treat diffusely sclerosed coronary and/or peripheral arteries, which is at present impossible; and 3) to open the artery in case of total occlusion and chronic stenosis.

Thus, laser angioplasty may be used on its own or in combination with either coronary artery bypass surgery or balloon angioplasty.

Laser treatment is still experimental. However, it appears to be very promising. In a section to follow, a model has been developed based on different possibilities of laser success as an alternative to CABG. As will be shown, these could have considerable health services system implications, especially for financial costs.

Table 1 Estimated Annual Expenses of Operating a Carbon Dioxide Laser Dedicated to Surgery, US Dollars

Technical Expenses	
Equipment[1]	$10-20,000
Maintenance	3-10,000
Other maintenance and remodelling	0-13,000
Technical staff[2]	20-40,000
Spare parts	1- 3,000
Total Expenses	$34-86,000
Expense per use (maximal)	$400
Expense per use (minimal)	$40

Note: These financial estimates are not based on actual experience with a laser, but are presented for illustration only. The method of estimation follows that used in calculating the expenses of operating a computed tomography (CT) scanner (51)

1) Based on an estimated price of US$50-100,000, amortized over a five year period.
2) Staff here excludes clinical staff, such as physicians and nurses, who presumably would already be providing these services or similar services. Staff referred to here are engineers, physicists, and so forth.

Scenarios. To illustrate the possible implications of laser developments on health care, scenarios were developed concerning successful laser treatment of coronary artery disease. These scenarios show the possible impacts of only one of the many possible applications of lasers in the future. On the other hand, these scenarios are only intended as illustrations. The outcomes given in this section are not predictions, although experts on lasers and on cardiology have agreed that they are within a reasonable set of possibilities.

Models Developed in the Scenario Commission on Cardiovascular Disease. For the purpose of examining the impact of lasers on coronary artery disease, a model of treatment of coronary artery disease was used. The STG commission study **The Heart of the Future, The Future of the Heart** (61) developed two models as part of its study: one on incidence and prevalence of ischemic heart disease and one on chronic care for ischemic heart disease. The rates of disease developed in the first model were used as inputs to the second model. The models were developed by Dr. Wilbert Wils, who modified it for this project. Details of the models can be found in the STG report.

The incidence and prevalence model is based on available data on rates of cardiovascular disease and ischemic heart disease. Figure 1 shows mortality in the Netherlands from ischemic heart disease over time. It can be seen that the mortality rate from ischemic heart disease in the Netherlands rose in both sexes until 1972. Since 1972, age-specific mortality has fallen. Mortality is taken as the principle indicator of the prevalence of chronic heart disease in the model. Figure 2 shows how under conservative assumptions age-adjusted mortality rates for ischemic heart disease decline to the year 2020. Incidence (those with the onset of the disease) also falls in the model. Hospital morbidity is still increasing at present, in part because of the aging of the population and higher rates of disease in older people, and in part because the onset of the clinical disease may be delayed for some time after the patient actually has the disease. The numbers of treatments such as coronary artery bypass graft are also still increasing because clinical capacity if still expanding and catching up with an accumulated backlog of patients needing treatment. The model is consistent with observed trends, and with clinical experience.

Twenty different scenarios were considered in the model. These include changing life-styles, changing acute care, and changing chronic care. Possible effects of lasers were not considered. In all scenarios, the age-dependent incidence of ischemic heart disease declines at least until 1995. Prevalence also falls, but more slowly. As shown in Figure 3, the rate of coronary artery bypass surgery falls much more rapidly under a variety of assumptions. As can be seen, the number of candidates for intervention falls in all scenarios at least to 1990. This decline is independent of the fall in age-specific incidence and mortality rates. It reflects a rapid resolution of the backlog of candidates for coronary artery bypass surgery, built up during the years that there was limited capacity for this surgery.

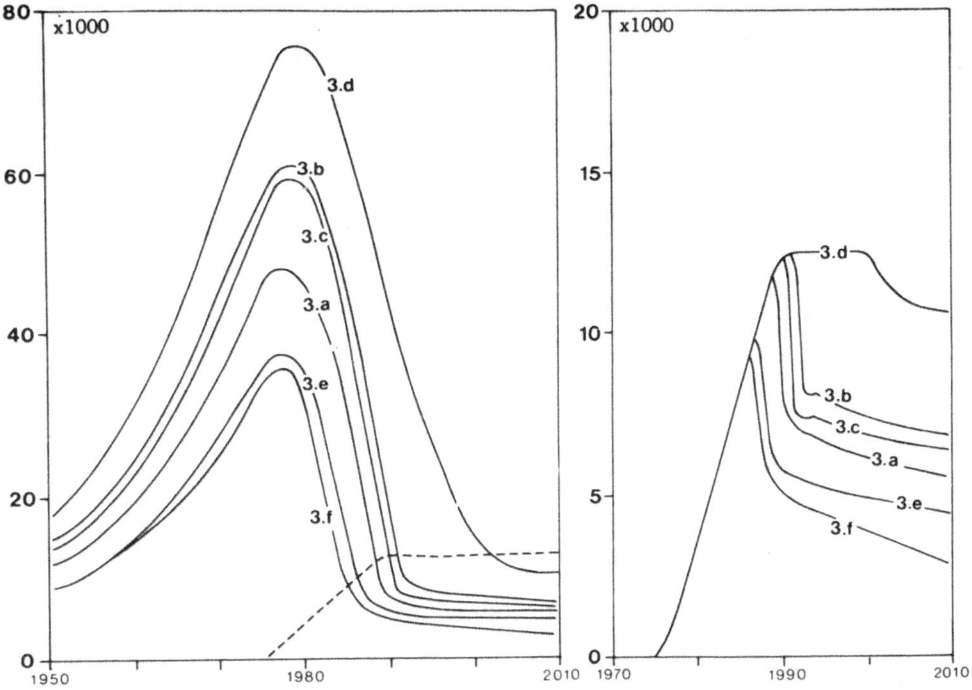

Candidates for coronary surgery coronary operations

--------- capacity for coronary operations

3.a: scenario 6 years - 6 years on average of satisfactory drug treatment
3.b: scenario 5 years - 5 years on average of satisfactory drug treatment,
3.c: scenario 5 years and relatively more PTCA
3.d: scenario 4 years and improved intervention in acute cases of Ischemic heart disease
3.e: scenario 7 years
3.f: scenario 7 years, relatively more PTCA, improved rehabilitation of Ischemic heart disease patients, and improvement of lifestyles

Figure 3 Bypass-operations and candidates for bypass operations following six scenarios for chronic care

Source: 61

Figure 4 shows the logic of the model for chronic care.* Starting from the upper left hand corner, healthy people become symptomatic with ischemic heart disease. They then become patients on medication (and some of those become healthy and move back into the healthy state). Of those people who are symptomatic and on medication, 7 percent a year have a medical examination that includes angiography to directly examine the state of their coronary arteries. Of that group, 55-60 percent continue on medical therapy, 5 percent have severe disease and leave the treatment model, and 35-40 percent have further intervention. Of those who continue on medication, 5 percent a year have further intervention.

Of the group receiving further intervention, 15-20 percent are candidates for PTCA and 80-85 percent are candidates for coronary artery bypass surgery. Of those having PTCA, 15-20 percent have immediate coronary artery bypass surgery and 80-85 percent join the group of post-PTCA patients. Of that group, 6 percent a year have a repeat PTCA procedure and 9 percent a year become candidates for coronary artery bypass. On average, PTCA helps a patient for about 4 years before some other procedure is necessary. Of those having coronary artery bypass surgery, 98 percent survive and join the group of post-coronary surgery patients. Of that group, 5 percent a year die and 5 percent a year must have a repeat coronary artery bypass graft. On average, coronary artery bypass graft helps a patient for 9 years before another procedure is needed. While coronary artery bypass is more effective in terms of the time between procedures, it is a more serious procedure, with higher morbidity and mortality and higher cost.

*) For a detailed description of the model, see the STG report on cardiovascular disease (61). This footnote presents a brief explanation of the Figure. The boxes represent groups of patients. The lines with arrows with 'valve' symbols (▷◁) represent flows of people between boxes or between boxes and 'outside of the model' (indicated by cloud-shaped figures). Those outside of the model include healthy people (those without symptoms of ischemic heart disease), persons severely handicapped by ischemic heart disease, and the deceased. The indicated percentages refer to an annual percentage outflow from the box that is the source of the flow or to distribution of parts of the flow to alternative states. These percentages are chosen in accordance with data from the medical literature or from expert estimates. Number should be seen as indicators of a range rather than as precise data. The conclusions are similarly limited.

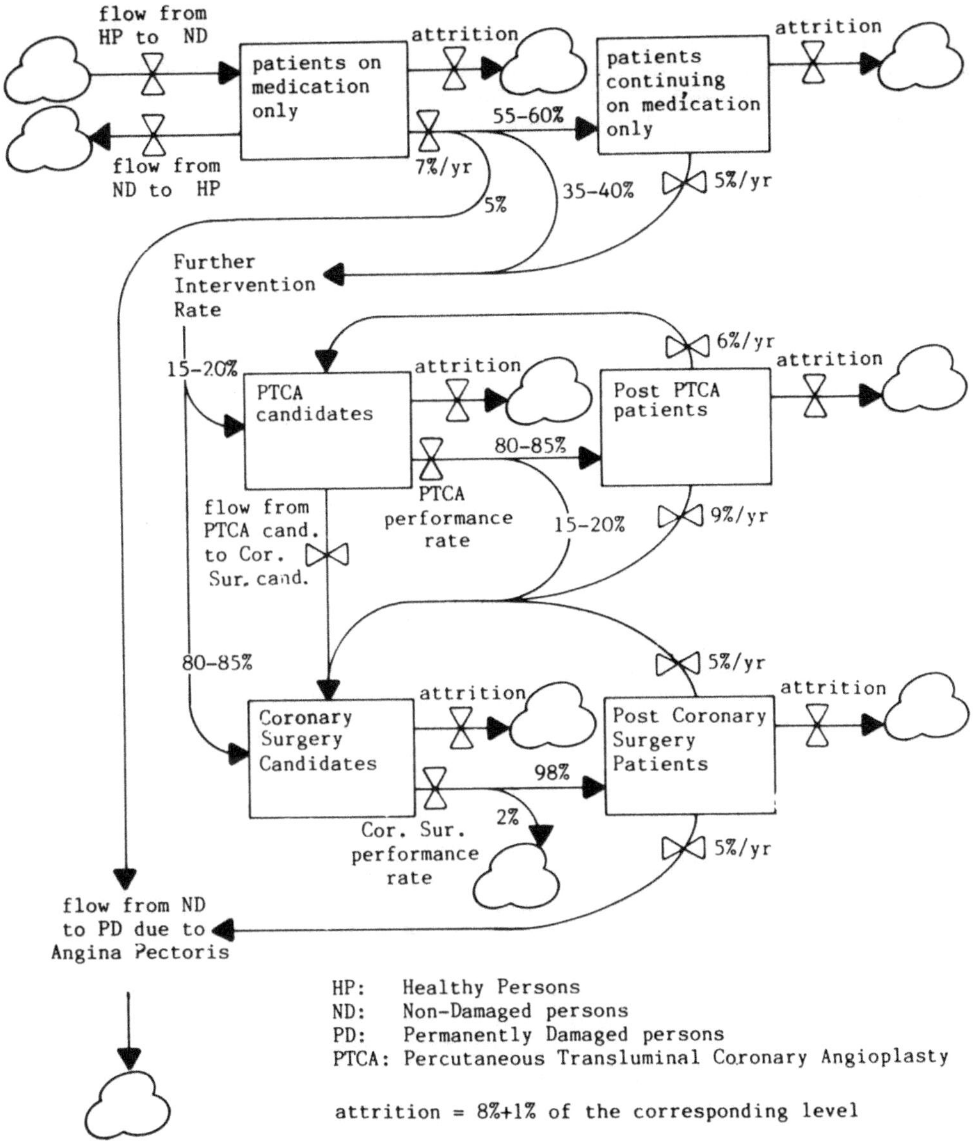

Figure 4 Structure of the Model for Chronic Care

Source: 61

Modifications of the Model for Chronic Care Made by the Project on Future Health Care Technology. The assumptions used in the model, and shown in Figure 4, reflect experience as reported in the scientific literature, supplemented by clinical experience in the Netherlands until 1984. Under the assumptions in the model, the number of PTCA procedures carried out in the Netherlands in 1984 was approximately 1,700. After 1984, the base scenario in the model assumed a slow increase in the number of PTCA procedures.

Experts in the field of treatment for coronary artery disease, asked to review this base case in 1986, stated that the situation has changed rapidly. In 1984, PTCA was used primarily for the treatment of people with narrowing or blockage of one coronary artery. More recently, however, many centers have begun to use PTCA with patients with stenosis (narrowing) of two or more arteries. Under the base case, the number of PTCA procedures in the model in the Netherlands in 1986 was still approximately 1.700. In reality, the number of PTCA procedures in the Netherlands was estimated to be about 2,600 in 1985 and 3,500 in 1986.

Data are not available to indicate how the assumptions of the chronic treatment model have changed since 1984. Therefore, different assumptions which experts considered realistic were used within the model and their effects examined. The model was found to be most sensitive to changes in the number of patients going on to further intervention (point 1 in the chronic care model) and to the percentage of those patients having PTCA instead of coronary artery bypass graft (point 2 in the chronic care model).

Therefore, two important changes were made in the chronic care model. One was to diminish the percentage of patients who receive prolonged medical treatment by assuming that 10 percent per year have further intervention (instead of 5 percent). (This change was made at point 1 in the chronic disease model.) The other change was to increase the percentage of PTCA procedures among those patients with further intervention (point 2 in the model) from 15-20 percent in 1980 to 35-40 percent in 1990 and beyond. These changes led to a level of PTCA procedures consistent with experience of 1985 and 1986.

These changes in the chronic disease model gave results consistent with PTCA experience during 1985 and 1986.

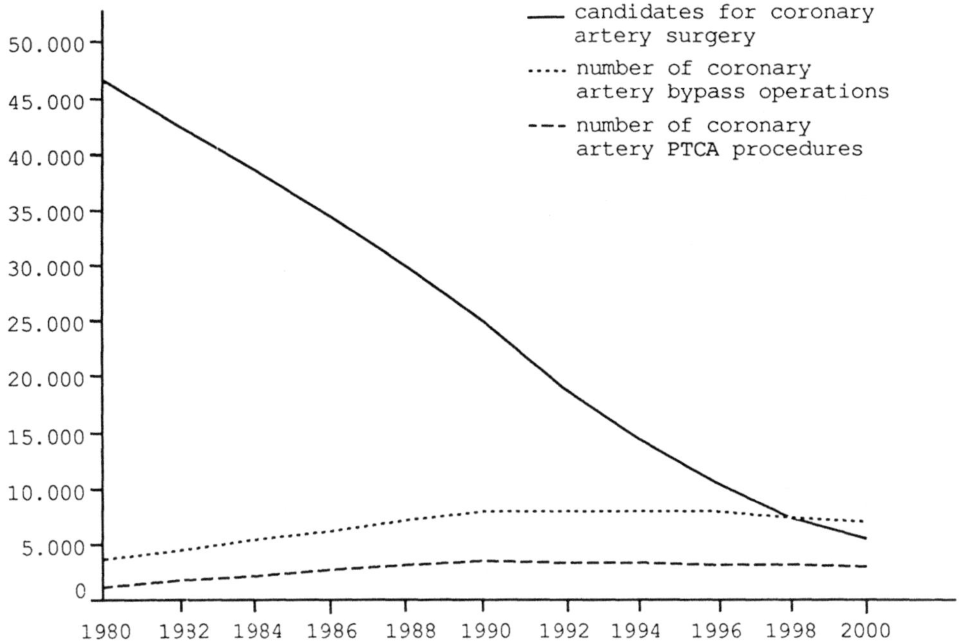

Figure 5 Scenario of the Base Case

Figure 5 shows graphically the results for the base case. It can be seen that the number of candidates for coronary artery surgery falls steadily because the backlog of candidates for surgery is cleared. At the same time, the number of coronary artery bypass operations increases until 1990 and then levels off, so that the number of candidates and the number of operations come into balance in the year 1998. This case continues the assumptions for PTCA success already described. In this scenario, in the year 2000 there would be 7,100 coronary artery bypass operations and 3,100 PTCA procedures.

Scenarios Considering Laser Applications in Coronary Disease. The laser raises the possibility of increasing the flow of patients to alternatives to coronary artery bypass graft (CABG). At this time, how the laser would be used is not entirely clear. It could be used alone or as part of a PTCA procedure. For example, the laser might burn away thrombus, making it possible to pass a balloon catheter through the blood vessel. The exact form of the ultimate procedure, however, does not matter in the model. What is important is the flow of patients into each box.

Alternative assumptions were chosen to examine future changes in chronic disease treatment and how they might be affected by successful laser therapy. These alternatives focused on increasing the number of patients going on to further intervention (point 1) and/or the percentage of those patients having PTCA instead of coronary artery bypass graft (point 2). In each of these alternative scenarios, effective laser therapy was assumed beginning in 1990. In all, 10 scenarios were developed. In addition, the percentages of those needing repeat procedures were altered, but these changes had limited impact on the overall results.

The scenario presented in Figure 6 assumes, because of laser success, a gradual change among those going to further intervention, to increase the percentage with a laser/PTCA procedure to 60 percent (point 2 in the model) in the year 2000. This might be a reasonable upper limit of the impact of effective laser therapy. In this case, the number of candidates falls more rapidly, and capacity for coronary artery bypass graft exceeds the number of candidates by 1998. The number of coronary artery bypass procedures also falls more rapidly after 1996 in this scenario. In this scenario, there would be 6,300 coronary artery bypass operations in the year 2000 and 4,500 laser/PTCA procedures.

The other scenarios each generated numbers similar to those presented. In all cases, laser effectiveness increases the number of PTCA/laser procedures by 1,500 to 1,700 and decreases the number of CABG procedures annually by about 800. Because of the similarity of the impact of laser effectiveness in all scenarios, they will not be presented here. They are available, however, to any interested reader. It should be noted, at the same time, that the alternate scenarios do indicate a large range of results for the numbers of CABG and PTCA procedures; these differences could be quite important for health planning purposes.

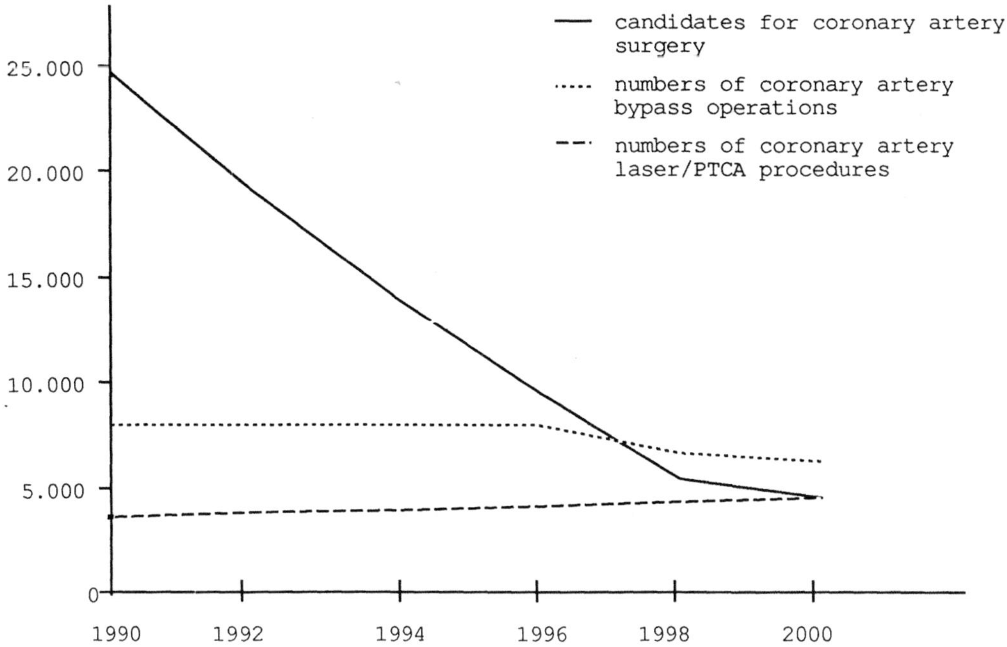

Figure 6 Scenario Following Introduction of Laser Angioplasty in 1990

Financial Estimates. Table 2 shows the financial implications of these differences. The cost of each procedure was taken from estimates in the STG report (61). The cost of a laser/PTCA procedure was assumed to be somewhat more than a PTCA procedure because of the capital investment in the laser. Coronary artery bypass graft is assumed to cost 25,000 guilders (including hospitalization), PTCA is assumed to cost 2,000 guilders (including 2 days of hospitalization), and laser/PTCA is assumed to cost 2,500 guilders.

These estimates are subject to many possible criticisms. First, they are not based on careful studies of costs, but are estimates based on

Table 2 Financial Costs of Alternate Scenarios in the Year 2000

Assumptions		Financial Costs
Cost of CABG	-	25,000 guilders
Cost of PTCA	-	2,000 guilders
Cost of laser/PTCA	-	2,500 guilders
Cost of Base Case	-	184 million guilders
Cost of Laser Success Case	-	169 million guilders
Difference (Saving)	-	15 million guilders

limited available data. Second, they do not take into account technological changes over time. Third, costs could vary dramatically from center to center and from country to country. Therefore, these estimates should only be considered indicative. They should **not** be taken as definitive.

The cost of coronary artery bypass graft and PTCA treatment in the base case in the year 2000 is 184 million guilders. The cost of coronary artery bypass graft and laser/PTCA treatment in the laser success case in the year 2000 is 169 million guilders. The difference is 15 million guilders. Perhaps more important is the potentially disruptive effects on the system, if surgeons, operating theatres, and operating teams are in excess.

The cost of the high technology case is almost the same as the base case because the small reduction in coronary artery bypass procedures balances the larger increase in laser/PTCA procedures.

Conclusions

The purpose of these scenarios is not to predict that this will in fact happen. The purpose is to show how one technological change can have potentially important consequences for the health care system. This case is particularly interesting because of the prevailing impression that the Netherlands needs more of a capability for doing coronary artery bypass graft. However, partially as a result of the

STG Commission Report on Cardiovascular Disease (61), the validity of plans based on extrapolation of past trends is already being questioned.

From these results, and from the Commission Report, it appears that the present supply of surgeons for performing coronary artery bypass grafts will be (at least) adequate in the future. Laser success could turn the perceived shortage into an obvious excess within a few years.

Section 4 – Conclusions

The use of laser in health care is rapidly evolving. Already, lasers are finding wide use in medicine, especially in certain areas of surgery. In the future, many more applications, including both diagnostic and therapeutic, will undoubtedly be demonstrated.

At the same time, one cannot automatically assume that any application is beneficial. Each must be carefully evaluated. This raises difficult problems of evaluation. For example, the laser needs to be evaluated in every form of surgery for which it has been proposed, in comparison with conventional surgical therapy.

This report has focused on treatment of coronary artery disease with lasers. Coronary disease is one of the most costly conditions for society, and more efficient and effective methods are very much needed. Lasers offer the possibility of a more effective treatment, associated with less pain for the patient and lower cost for society. However, this application must also be carefully evaluated.

The application of lasers in the health care system promises to cause or stimulate important changes in the organization of care. For example, patterns of specialization will change, as certain physicians become intensive users of lasers. The need for general surgeons may very well fall.

In several areas of medicine, particularly in surgery, lasers offer potential financial savings. However, for these savings to be realized, other investments and expenditures must be foregone. In particular, the number of operating rooms, hospital beds, and surgeons could possibly be decreased. This potential is particularly pertinent at a time when planners are projecting a need for increased numbers of surgeons and operating rooms.

Lasers will certainly raise difficult issues of planning and policy during the next few years. Potential investment in lasers for health care purposes is truly enormous. Lasers can improve care, and perhaps even lower health care costs in many areas. However, if decisions are made without the benefit of careful evaluative studies, investments in lasers could drive up health care costs without corresponding benefit.

Conclusion 1. The government of the Netherlands and other policy making bodies need to monitor the situation with laser applications in health care

Little is known presently about the number of lasers in the Netherlands or how they are used. In short, there is no basis for future planning. The first task is to develop simple base-line information. Over time, policy makers will need better information on evolving technological trends with lasers, as well as data on use in the Netherlands. Data on efficacy, safety, and cost-effectiveness of various laser applications will also be needed.

Conclusion 2. Expertise on lasers is needed in the Netherlands

An active, organized research program on medical applications of lasers would be beneficial for the Netherlands. At present, there are few activities, and they are scattered, disorganized, and under-funded. Training programs are needed to develop both clinical and technical expertise with lasers.

It is particularly important to make evaluation a key part of any approach to lasers. Future decisions need to be based on sound information on efficacy, safety, financial costs, and implications for the health care system. At the same time, the many applications of lasers in health care are beyond the capability of a country such as the Netherlands to evaluate. International cooperation could be very beneficial. The World Health Organization and the European Community (EC) are both interested in evaluating lasers. With some encouragement, it could be possible to develop a truly international effort.

One specific suggestion is to develop a national center concerned with laser applications in health care. As mentioned above, present activities are fragmented. There is no focus of expertise for development, evaluation, or advice. However, such a center could only be beneficial if it were multidisciplinary in nature. Physicists and other scientists familiar with the technical aspects of lasers, as well as clinical expertise, are needed. Incorporating epidemiological and statistical expertise in such a center for the purposes of evaluative studies could also be beneficial. However, this is only one option for reaching the goal defined in this section. This project did not have the capability of evaluating this option.

Conclusion 3. Increased involvement of Dutch industry in medical applications of lasers could be beneficial

Dutch industry is not substantially involved in medical applications of lasers. Yet Dutch companies are involved with lasers - the technological capability is available. Dutch industry could be encouraged to explore this rapidly growing area.

In the future, policy makers will need to deal effectively with many dimensions of laser applications. Research and evaluation need to be fostered. Capital investments will need to be made. Controls need to be developed for laser use. Organized standards will be necessary for lasers. Training is necessary. Payment for services based on lasers will need to be developed where appropriate.

Laser applications in health care raise many important implications for the future.

Appendixes

APPENDIX A TECHNICAL BACKGROUND ON LASERS

Laser devices employ an energizing source or pump, such as high-intensity light or electric current, to cause atoms, molecules, or ions in a medium to radiate highly directional light of (almost) a single wavelength, called coherent light (See Figure 7). (The term 'wavelength' refers to the electromagnetic spectrum, which is made up of radiation ranging from radio waves with long wavelengths and low frequencies to gamma rays with short wavelenghts and high frequencies.)

Atoms and molecules exist in nature at low and high energy levels. An atom or molecule can be 'excited' to a higher energy level by an external energy source. When an atom returns to a lower energy level, it can give off a photon. An ordinary light source gives off photons at many different wavelengths, which move in different directions. (The range or band of the wavelengths is referred to as bandwidth.)

In lasers, the wavelength varies with the nature of the medium selected. The medium may be solid, liquid, or gaseous, for example, ruby, organic dyes, or carbon dioxide. The medium is excited by the energy source. Excited atoms begin to give up photons. The photons radiate in all directions: much of this radiation is dissipated in the form of heat. A small percentage of the photons travel along the axis of the laser cavity. When one of these photons passes by another energized atom, it stimulates that atom to give up energy in the form of an identical photon, which moves in the same direction. The process continues until a stream of photons, all having the same wavelength and moving in the same direction, travels the length of the medium (see Figure 7).

As they move through the laser cavity, the photons bounce between two mirrors, one a full mirror, the other a partially transmitting mirror that allows some of the light waves to escape. The photons build up between the two mirrors, and the fraction of light that escapes forms a single beam of intense coherent light. The light can be transmitted through a series of mirrors to an operating microscope, through an articulating arm, or may be focused on the end of a small flexible quartz rod called a fiber. Endoscopes are now made from such quartz rods (fiberoptic endoscopes), which allows transmission of laser energy through endoscopic devices.

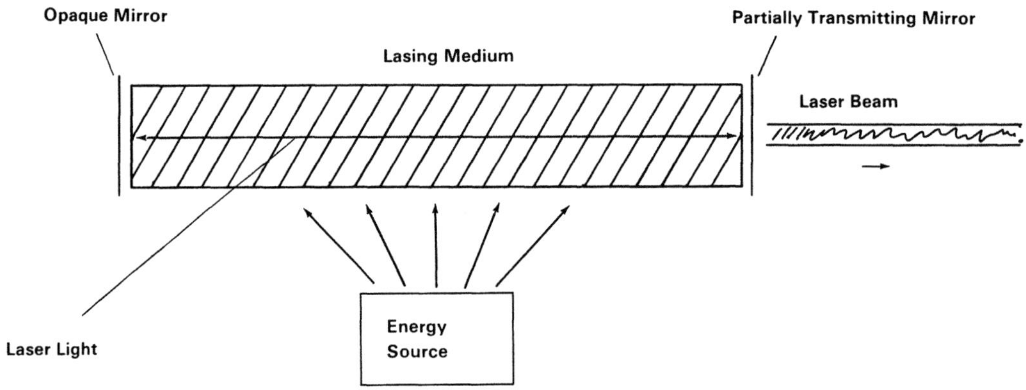

Figure 7 How a Laser Works

Lasers can be designed to generate light in pulses or continuously (continuous wave, or cw). Some lasers can be tuned over a range of wavelengths. The power of the laser beam can be low (referred to as 'soft' lasers) or high, as in weapons.

Presently available lasers using carbon dioxide operate within the infrared spectrum. (See Table 3). In the near-infrared spectrum, there are neodymium-doped glass, neodymium-doped yttrium aluminum garnet (YAG or Nd-YAG), and other lasers. The argon ion laser produces light in the blue-green region of the spectrum. Several types of ion lasers are used in the region of visible light.

Pulsed, ultraviolet-emitting excimer lasers are being used experimentally. The term 'excimer' is derived from 'excited dimer', where dimer refers to a molecule comprising two atoms of the same species. Excimer lasers can be made with rare gases such as xenon, krypton, and argon, and from rare gases in association with a halide, such as fluoride or bromide.

However, there are needs for other types of lasers. For example, there is no laser that produces light in the visible range with relatively high power. Such lasers could be used in large-screen displays. A free electron laser has been described that can be tuned across all laser wavelenghts at high-power, but this laser requires a linear accelerator. Perhaps in the future the falling cost of such a laser will make it practical, at least in large medical centers (19).

Table 3 Some Commonly Used Lasers in Health Care

Name	Wavelength um	Use
Carbon dioxide	10.6	tissue vaporization
Neodymium - Yttrium Aluminium Garnet (Nd-YAG)	1.06	sealing by heat shrinkage
Argon	0.5	photocoagulation
Argon-ion driven Rhodamine dye	0.63	differential chemical destruction
Helium neon	0.63	aiming beam for CO_2 and YAG lasers; used to measure blood flow

Source: Reference (18).

APPENDIX B METHOD FOR THIS REPORT

The need for examining future health care technology was recognized by the Dutch Steering Committee on Future Health Scenarios (STG) in 1984. (The STG is an independent advisory group to the Dutch government set up in 1983 to carry out scenario studies as an aid to long-term health planning). The STG initiated the Project on Future Health Care Technology. The World Health Organization, European Office (EURO), agreed to support the project financially and logistically.

The project had two specific objectives:
1. To identify future technological developments in health care, with brief descriptions of potential technologies; and
2. To carry out prospective assessments of four high priority technologies or areas of technological development.

The project began in April 1985. A Commission on Future Health Care Technology made up of 10 members and 5 official observers was appointed to guide the project. Surveys of experts were carried out in the United States and Europe. The information from the surveys, supplemented by material from the scientific literature and from interviews, was the basis for the overall descriptions of health care technology. The assistance of these many individuals and groups is specifically acknowledged in appendixes to Volumes 1 and 2 of this report.

A detailed description of methods for the entire project is presented in an appendix to Volume 1 of the series. An updated version may be found in Volume 2. And each case study contains a methods description specific to that case.

The project plan called for four technologies to be prospectively assessed. In September 1985, the Commission met and endorsed four cases:
1. implications of neurosciences;
2. biotechnology - probably examining both monoclonal antibodies and vaccines;
3. laser applications, especially in surgery and in the treatment of vascular disease, especially coronary artery disease; and
4. genetic testing and diagnosis.

Later, with funding from the Ministry of Economic Affairs, medical imaging and home care technology were also developed as case studies.

A draft report on lasers in medicine was written with the assistance of Dr. Martin van Gemert of St. Joseph Ziekenhuis in Eindhoven. The paper was then circulated to a group of experts who met on 10 June 1986 to discuss it (see front of report for group members). The group also helped develop a number of plausible alternative assumptions about the future impact of lasers on coronary artery surgery. The STG report on the future of coronary disease had developed a model on the future of coronary artery bypass surgery and percutaneous transluminal coronary angioplasty. The assumptions on the future of lasers were used in this model to project different possible scenarios for the impact of lasers on coronary artery surgery (as described in this report). The model was developed with the strong assistance of Dr. Wilbert Wils. During the summer, the model was elaborated and the first complete draft of the report finalized.

In a meeting of 24 September 1986, the Commission discussed the draft report on lasers. Suggestions for conclusions on the laser case were incorporated into the report with other changes suggested by reviewers. The findings of the model and the draft conclusions of the report were submitted to the Commission in its meeting of 20 November 1986. Further suggestions were made by the Commission. The report was then revised, sent to reviewers for comments, and revised again. It was approved by the Commission at its meeting of 4 February 1987 and was submitted to the STG in mid-March 1987.

APPENDIX C GLOSSARY OF TERMS

Acute: In medical care, used to describe a condition that has a sudden onset, sharp rise, and short course (compare **Chronic**).

Ambulatory care: Medical services provided to patients who are not hospitalized.

Angina: Any spasmodic, choking, or suffocative pain. The term is often used to denote angina pectoris--a condition characterized by severe, transient chest pain, accompanied by a feeling of suffocation and impending death, that is due to a deficiency in the supply of oxygen to the heart.

Angiography: See **Arteriography**.

Arteriography: Visualization of an artery using X-radiographs after the injection of radiopaque (impervious to the rays) material into the bloodstream. Angiography is the same except refers to visualization in this fashion of any blood vessel.

Arteriosclerosis: A condition in which the arterial walls become thickened and hardened. The causes are multiple and complex, and often incompletely known. Also called 'hardening of the arteries'. See **Atherosclerosis**.

Atherosclerosis: A very common form of arteriosclerosis in which deposits of fibrous and cellular tissue, cholesterol, and fat accumulate in large and medium-sized arteries, impeding blood flow.

Balloon dilatation: Using a balloon attached to a catheter to dilate or open blocked blood vessels. The catheter is passed through the blood vessels to the site of blockage and the balloon is inflated.

Biopsy: The removal and examination, usually microscopic, of tissue from the living body, performed to establish precise diagnosis.

Bronchoscopy: Examining the bronchi (tubes in the lungs) by endoscope.

Cancer: A cellular tumor, the natural course of which is fatal. Cancers are divided into two broad categories, carcinoma and sarcoma.

Carcinogenic: Causing cancer.

Carcinoma: One of the two broad categories of cancer. Carcinoma can be categorized according to the type of cells in which it orignates. For example, an epithelioma originates in epithelial cells (cells of the skin). A basal cell carinoma originates in basal cells of the skin.

Cardiac catheterization: Passage of a small catheter through a vein or artery into the heart for purposes of securing blood samples, determining intracardiac pressures, and detecting cardiac anomalies.

Cardiac radionuclide imaging: The imaging of the heart by the detection of radioactivity in the heart muscle or heart chambers following the injection of a radionuclide or radiopharmaceutical.

Cardiovascular: Pertaining to the heart and blood vessels.

Cataract: A loss of transparency of the lens of the eye or of its capsule.

Cholesterol: A steroid alcohol present in animal cells and body fluids, important in physiological processes and implicated as a factor in atherosclerosis.

Chromosome: In animal and human cells, a threadlike structure that carries genetic information arranged in a linear sequence. It consists of a complex of nucleic acids and proteins.

Chronic: Lingering, lasting, as opposed to acute. A term used to describe persistent disease.

Clinical Trial: An experiment carried out for the purpose of evaluating the efficacy and safety of a health care technology. The nature of the control group is a critical issue in a clinical trial. See **Control group, Randomized clinical trial.**

Colposcope: An optical device used to examine and photograph the vagina and cervix. Using dyes and other techniques, it is possible to identify pre-malignant and malignant changes in the cells of these tissues.

Continuous wave laser: A laser in which the 'pumping' energy is applied continually, giving rise to continuous production of laser light. See **Pulsed laser.**

Control group: In a randomized clinical trial, the group receiving no treatment or some treatment with which the group receiving experimental treatment is compared. The control treatment is generally a standard treatment, a placebo, or no treatment. Compare **Experimental group.**

Coronary angiography: See **Coronary arteriography.**

Coronary arteries: Arteries that supply blood to the heart.

Coronary arteriography: Arteriography of the coronary arteries.

Coronary artery bypass graft (CABG) surgery: A surgical procedure in which a vein or an artery is used to bypass a constricted portion of one or more coronary arteries. This procedure has become the primary surgical approach to the treatment of coronary artery disease.

Coronary artery disease (coronary heart disease): Narrowing or blockage of the coronary arteries, which usually results in reduced blood flow to the heart muscle.

Coronary heart disease: See **Coronary artery disease.**

Cost-benefit analysis (CBA): An analytical technique that compares the costs of a project or technological application to the resultant benefits, with both costs and benefits expressed by the same measure. This measure is nearly always monetary.

Cost-effectiveness analysis (CEA): An analytical technique that compares the costs of a project or of alternative projects to the resultant benefits, with costs and benefits/effectiveness expressed by different measures. Costs are usually expressed in dollars, but benefits/effectiveness are ordinarily expressed in terms such as 'lives saved', 'disability avoided', 'quality-adjusted life years saved', or any other relevant objectives.

Cost-effectiveness analysis/cost-benefit analysis (CEA/CBA): A composite term used to refer to a family of analytical techniques that are employed to compare costs and benefits of programs or technologies. Literally, as used at OTA, the term means 'cost-effectiveness analysis/cost-benefit analysis'.

Cytofluorometry: Studying cells using fluorescent material to 'tag' them.

Dermatology: The specialty of medicine dealing with the skin.

DNA: Deoxyribonucleic acid. The nucleic acid in chromosomes that codes for genetic information.

Doppler: The term refers to the phenomenon of the pitch of sound being higher when the object is approaching the listener, as is obvious with a locomotive whistle. The phenomenon is used to study blood flow in arteries (and sometimes in veins) and in the heart.

Echocardiography: A method of imaging the heart walls and internal structures of the heart by the echo obtained from beams of ultrasonic waves directed through the heart wall.

Effectiveness: Same as efficacy (see below) except that it refers to '...average or actual conditions of use'.

Efficacy: The probability of benefit to individuals in a defined population from a medical technology applied for a given medical problem under ideal conditions of use.

Electrocardiogram (EKG or ECG): A graphic tracing of the changes of electrical potential of the heart occurring during each heartbeat; usually performed with the patient supine and at rest.

Endarterectomy: Surgical removal of the inner layer of an artery when the artery is thickened and obstructed.

Endoscope: An instrument used for the examination of the interior of a canal or hollow organ. Endoscopes are frequently used to examine the gastrointestinal tract and the respiratory organs (lungs and bronchi). (See **Fiberoptics**).

Epidemiology: The scientific study of the distribution and occurrence of human diseases and health conditions, and their determinants.

Epidemiologic studies: Studies concerned with the relationships of various factors determining the frequency and distribution of specific diseases in a human community.

Excimer laser: The term 'excimer' is derived from 'excited dimer', where a dimer refers to a molecule made up of two atoms of the same species. Excimer lasers can be made using rare gases (xenon, krypton, and argon). They are also made using rare gases in association with a halide (such as fluoride or bromide). Excimer lasers produce ultraviolet light waves.

Exercise tolerance testing (exercise stress testing): Testing the response of the heart to exercise while observing the ECG and other physiological functions of the heart.

Experimental group: In a randomized clinical trial, the group receiving the treatment being evaluated for safety and efficacy. The experimental treatment may be a new technology, an existing technology applied to a new problem, or an accepted treatment about whose safety or efficacy there is doubt. Compare **Control group**.

Extra-corporeal shock wave lithotrypsy (ESWL): The use of sound waves from outside the body to break up stones, especially of the urinary tract.

Fallopian tube: The oviduct, the tube which connects the overies to the uterus and through which the ovum travels.

Fiberoptics: Having to do with sight through glass fibers. Fiberoptics in health care are primarily used with endoscopes (scopes for looking into the body) made up of bundles of glass fibers, along with hollow channels for passage of air, water, and instruments. One bundle of fibers transmits light to the site, and the other transmits the image of the illuminated object or body part to the other end of the endoscope. The fiberoptic endoscope can be bent or curved without distorting the image.

Flow cytometry: A method of studying cells used primarily as a research tool, but now, with automated systems and other advances, spreading rapidly into routine application. The cells are in a fluid and flow past a fixed point where they are studied by some method, for example, by their light-scattering properties. Flow cytometry is increasingly using monoclonal antibodies, and lasers are being developed as a part of such systems.

Flow cytofluorometry: Similar to flow cytometry, but involving tagging cells with fluorescent material.

Flow karyometric methods: Similar to flow cytometry, but used to examine the nucleus of cells, focusing particularly on chromosomal structure.

Fluorescence: The property of rendering certain light visible (e.g. ultraviolet) or of becoming self-luminous when exposed to light rays.

Glaucoma: A disease due to increase of the fluids of the eyeball, raising pressure and causing damage to the eye structures.

Hemodynamic: Relating to the blood circulation.

Hemorrhage: The escape of blood from the blood vessels, either into surrounding tissues or into the environment.

Hemorrhagic: Of or pertaining to a copious discharge of blood from the blood vessels.

Hologram: A three-dimensional picture made on a photographic film or plate without the use of a camera and consisting of a pattern of interference produced by a split coherent beam of light.

Iatrogenic: Resulting from the activities of physicians. The term is commonly applied to infections, drug reactions, or other mishaps that occur while patients are hospitalized.

Immunology: The scientific study of immunity, induced sensitivity, and allergy.

Incidence: The frequency of new occurrences of disease within a defined time interval. Incidence rate is the number of new cases of specified disease divided by the number of people in a population over a specified period of time, usually 1 year. Compare **Prevalence**.

Infarct: An area of necrosis (death) of tissue, resulting from the obstruction of blood supply.

Innovation: In the context of medical devices, any product or product modification that substantially improves the quality or decreases the cost of a product, while introducing a technology, material, or concept not previously found in any similar product on the market. Also, something perceived to be new.

Inpatient care: Care that includes an overnight stay in a medical facility.

Ischemia: Insufficient blood supply to meet the full physiologic needs of the tissue for oxygen (but short of the degree of ischemia that results in necrosis).

Ischemic heart disease: Coronary artery disease of sufficient severity to result in angina pectoris or myocardial infarction.

Laparotomy: Surgical incision through the abdomen.

Laser: An instrument that produces a highly focussed, high power source of energy.

Length of stay (LOS): The number of days a patient remains in the hospital from admission to discharge.

Lesion: Any abnormal discontinuity of tissue or loss of function. A wound, injury, or one of the individual points or patches of a multifocal disease.

Lymphatic vessel: Vessels in the body in which the lymph, a clear yellowish fluid, circulates.

Malignant: Applied to cancer, resistant to treatment or tending to grow worse or recur after removal. Malignant cancers often spread both locally and through the blood stream. See **Metastasis**.

Medical device: Any instrument, apparatus, or similar or related article that is intended to prevent, diagnose, mitigate, or treat disease or to affect the structure or function of the body.

Medical imaging: The field involved in making images, or pictures, of the inside of the human body. Traditionally, imaging was done by x-ray, but a number of new devices have been developed or are being developed that do not use x-ray.

Medical technology: The drugs, devices, and medical and surgical procedures used in medical care, and the organizational and support systems within which such care is provided.

Melanoma: A kind of cancer of the skin, a pigmented mole.

Metastasis: In cancer, the appearance of cancer in parts of the body remote from the place of the primary tumor. Metastases are spread by the blood or lymph systems.

Mode locked laser: Mode-locking is only possible in lasers oscillating in many (longitudinal) modes. A fast switch inside the laser cavity is opened only at time intervals corresponding to the round-trip time of a photon in the laser cavity. This process is called 'mode-locking'. It leads to very short pulses (in the picosecond range) of high power laser light. Mode-locking can be done in both continuous-wave and Q-switched lasers. See **Q-switched**.

Molecule: The smallest possible quantity of a substance that can exist independently and still retain the properties of the substance of which it forms a part. It is formed by a combination of two or more atoms.

Morbidity: The condition of being diseased.

Mortality rate: The death rate, often made explicit for a particular characteristic, e.g., age, sex, or specific cause of death. A mortality rate contains three essential elements: 1) the number of people in a population group exposed to the risk of death; 2) a time factor; 3) the number of deaths occurring in the exposed population during a certain time period.

Myocardial infarction: The death of muscle tissue of the heart due to blockage of a coronary artery or arteries.

Necrosis: Death of tissue.

Nevus (pl. nevi): A congenital mark or discolored patch of the skin due to pigmentation of the blood vessels.

Noninvasive technique: A technique that does not involve the penetration (by surgery or hypodermic needle) of the skin. Usually the term refers to diagnostic procedures.

Nonischemic heart disease: Heart disease from causes other than coronary artery disease (e.g., congenital heart disease, myocardiopathy).

Occlusion: In the context of the vascular system, the blocking off or obstruction of blood flow through a vessel.

Ophthalmology: The specialty of medicine dealing with the eye.

Organelle: One of the major fractions of the interior of a cell, including the nucleus, pieces of the cell membrance, and the mitochondria.

Outpatient care: Care that is provided in a hospital and that does not include an overnight stay.

Palliative treatment: Treatment designed to provide relief from a disease or condition (e.g., to provide comfort or reduce pain), but not to cure the disease or condition.

Pap smear: A type of smear of cells used particularly in cancer screening. Named after Papanicolaou, the inventor.

Pathogenesis: The mode of origin and development of a disease process.

Percutaneous transluminal coronary angioplasty (PTCA): A procedure in which a balloon tipped catheter is passed through a site of narrowing of the artery and theused balloon is inflated to reduce the obstruction.

Perforation: Being pierced with one or more holes.

Photon: A particle of light, a quantum of light.

Photocoagulation: Use of light to produce coagulation (or clotting).

Photosensitization: The use of light to activate compounds that are sensitive to light. It is being used experimentally in cancer treatment.

Plasma: The liquid portion of the blood in which particulate components of the blood are suspended.

Porphyrin: A biological compound commonly found in nature. Porphyrins can combine with different metals, which makes them important in certain bodily functions.

Posterior capsule: A tough lining of the back of the lens. It is usually left in the eye when a cataract is removed and has a tendency to become opaque (to not transmit light).

Premalignant: Precancerous. A lesion or tumor that is expected to turn to cancer after a time.

Prevalence: In epidemiology, the number of cases of disease, infected persons, or persons with disabilities or some other condition, present at a particular time and in relation to the size of the population. Also called 'prevalence rate'. Compare **Incidence**.

Procedure (medical or surgical): A medical technology involving any combination of drugs, devices, and provider skills and abilities. Appendectomy, for example, may involve at least drugs (for anesthesia), monitoring devices, surgical devices, and the skilled actions of physicians, nurses, and support staffs.

Psoriasis: A skin disease consisting of an eruption of rounded red patches with white scales which occur chiefly on the elbows, knees, scalp, and back.

Pulsed laser: If 'pumping' energy is applied intermittently in a laser, the laser light is produced in pulses. See **Continuous wave laser**.

Q-switched: A fast shutter can be placed in the laser cavity. When the shutter is closed, laser action is prevented and large numbers of excited atoms build up. When the shutter is opened, the energy stored is released in the form of a short (a few nanoseconds) and high-power light pulse. This is called a 'Q-switched laser'.

Random allocation: In a randomized clinical trial, allocation of individuals to treatment groups such that each individual has an equal probability of being assigned to any group.

Randomized clinical trial (RCT): An experiment designed to test the safety and efficacy of a medical technology in which people are randomly allocated to experimental or control groups, and outcomes are compared.

Recanalization: The process of opening a blockage, for example of a blood vessel, to make a new 'canal'.

Restenosis: Closing or narrowing again. Becoming stenosed again. Used to indicate the closing of a blood vessel that has opened surgically or with a balloon.

Retina: A delicate tissue consisting of several layers of cells behind the lens of the eye which contains the light-receptor cells and transmitting the signals from the outer world to the brain, thus bringing about sight.

Risk: A measure of the probability of an adverse or untoward outcome and the severity of the resultant harm to health of individuals in a defined population and associated with the use of a medical technology applied for a given medical problem under specified conditions of use.

RNA (ribonucleic acid): The nucleic acid found mainly in the nucleolus and ribosomes of the cell and associated with the control of cellular chemical activities.

Safety: A judgment of the acceptability of risk in a specified situation. See also **Risk**.

Saphenous vein: A vein (blood vessel) in the leg used in making bypasses of blocked blood vessels.

Sarcoma: One of the two main types of cancer.

Sclerosis: Hardening from chornic inflammation. Especially, the buildup of fibrous connective tissue.

Semi-conductor laser: A laser in which an excess of excited states of electrons are injected into the gap of a semi-conductor device (a diode or transister).

Somatic: A term used to refer to body tissues apart from reproductive (germinal) tissues.

Spectroscope: An instrument for resolving a ray of light from a body into its spectrum and for the observation of the spectrum. The spectroscope can carry out fine chemical and physical analyses of matter.

Stenosis: Narrowing.

Technology: The application of organized knowledge to practical ends.

Technology assessment: In general, a comprehensive form of policy research that examines the technical, economic, and social consequences of technological applications. It is especially concerned with unintended, indirect, or delayed social impacts. In health policy, however, the term more often is used to mean any form of policy analysis concerned with medical technology, especially the evaluation of efficacy and safety. The comprehensive form of technology assessment is then termed 'comprehensive technology assessment'.

Technology diffusion: The diffusion or spread of a medical technology into the health care system. It is generally thought to be in two phases: the initial phase in which decisions are made to adopt or reject the technology, and a subsequent phase in which decisions are made to use the technology.

Thrombolytic: Lysing or dissolving a thrombus.

Thrombosis: The formulation, development, or presence of a solid mass in a blood vessel or in the heart. It is composed of fibrin, platelets, and, in most instances, erythrocytes.

Ulcerated plaques: Breaks in the yellowish plaque formed within the intima and inner media (innermost and middle coats of the blood vessels) of large and medium-sized veins.

Vaporized: Converted from a solid to a liquid.

Vas deferens: The secretory duct of the testicle, which carries the sperm.

Ventricle: A small cavity. Most commonly, the term is used to refer to the two ventricles of the heart. The left ventricle is the chamber from which blood is pumped to the aorta and then to the arteries (and therefore to the tissues of the body). The right ventricle is the chamber from which blood that has returned to the heart is pumped to the lungs to be oxygenated.

Ventricular angiogram: A radiologic image of the ventricles of the heart obtained following the injection of a contrast dye.

Ventriculography: Imaging of the ventricles of the heart.

Vitreous humor: A jelly-like substance filling the interior of the eyeball behind the lens.

Wavelength: The length of the waves of any form of radiation, from radio waves with long wavelengths to gamma rays with short wavelengths.

APPENDIX D REFERENCES

1. Abela GS, Fenech A, Crea F, Conti CR. 'Hot tip': another method of laser vascular recanalization. Lasers in Surgery and Medicine 1985: 5: 327-335.

2. Abela GS, Normann SJ, Cohen DM et al. Laser recanalization of occluded atherosclerotic arteries in vivo and in vitro. Circulation 1985; 71: 403-411.

3. American College of Physicians. Percutanous transluminal angioplasty. Annals of Internal Medicine 1983; 99: 864-869.

4. Argon laser therapy opens new vista for early treatment of macular edema. Clinical Laser Monthly 1986; 4: 11-12.

5. Ascher P. Ten years of laser neurosurgery. Lasers in Medical Science 1986; 1: 298.

6. Borst C, Verdaasdonk RM, Smits P, WIld D, Rienks R, Jambroes G, Berengoltz SN, Robles de Medina EO, Hitchcock JF. Laser angioplasty with sapphire contact probe (abstract). Proceedings of the 1st International Symposium on Lasers in Cardiovascular Diseases, Vienna, 1986: 6.

7. Bowker TJ. Laser-tissue interaction and arterial perforation threshold in laser angioplasty. Seminars in Interventional Radiology 1986; 3: 39-46.

8. Bowker TJ, Cross FW, Rumsby PT, Gower MC, Rickards AF, Bown SG. Excimer laser angioplasty: quantitative comparison in vitro of three ultraviolet wavelengths on tissue ablation and haemolysis. Lasers in Medical Science 1986: 1: 91-101.

9. Carruth JAS, McKenzie AL. Medical lasers, science and clinical practice. Boston: Adam Hilger Ltd., 1986.

10. Choy DSJ, Stertzer SH, Rotterdam HZ, Bruno MS: Laser coronary angioplasty: experience with 9 cadaver hearts. American Journal of Cardiology 1982; 50, 1209-1211.

11. Choy DSJ, Stertzer SH, Rotterdam HZ, Sharrock N, Kaminow IP. Transluminal laser catheter angioplasty. American Journal of Cardiology 1982; 50: 1206-1208.

12. Choy DSJ, Stertzer SH, Myler RK, Marco J, Fournial G. Human coronary laser recanalization. Clinical Cardiology 1984; 7: 377-381.

13. Crea F, Davies G, McKenna W, Pashazade M, Taylor K, Maseri A. Percutaneous laser recanalization of coronary arteries. Lancet 1986; 2: 214-215.

14. Cumberland DC, Sanborn TA, Tayler DI, Moore DJ, Welsh CL, Greenfield AJ, Guben JK, Ryan TJ. Percutaneous laser thermal angioplasty, initial clinical results with a laser probe in total peripheral artery occlusions. Lancet 1986; 1: 1457-1459.

15. Cumberland DC, Starkey IR, Oakley GDG, Fleming JS, Smith GH, Goiti DI, Tayler JD. Percutaneous laser-assisted coronary angioplasty (letter). Lancet 1986; 2: 214.

16. Cumberland DC, Tayler DI, Procter AE. Laser-assisted percutaneous angioplasty: initial clinical experience in peripheral arteries. Clinical Radiology 1986; (in press).

17. Deckelbaum L, Donaldson RF, Isner JM, Bernstein J, Clarke RH. Elimination of pathologic injury associated with laser induced tissue ablation using pulsed energy delivery at low repetition rates. Journal of the Americal College of Cardiology 1985; 5: 408.

18. Department of Health and Social Security. Health equipment information. Number 141. Health technology assessment. London, May 1985.

19. Dixon JA. Lasers in surgery. Current Problems in Surgery 1984; 21: (entire issue).

20. van Erp WRM, Krepel VM. Percutane transluminale angioplastiek van bekken- en beenarterien. Thesis, University of Limburg, 1985 (ISBN 90-9000914-0).

21. Fourrier JF. Angioplasty by contact sapphire: in-vitro studies and clinical results. Presented at the 3rd Congress of the European Laser Association, Amsterdam, 6-8 November 1986.

22. Fowler CG. Fibrescopy Nd-YAG laser treatment of superficial bladder cancer. Lasers in Medical Sciences 1986; 1: 288 (abstract).

23. Fuller TA. Mid-infrared fiber optics. Lasers in Surgery and Medicine 1986; 6: 399-403.

24. van Gemert MJC., Berenbaum MC, Gijsberg GHM. Wavelength and light-dose dependence in tumour phototherapy with haematoporphyrin derivative. British Journal of Cancer 1985; 52: 43-49.

25. van Gemert MJC., Schets GACM, Stassen EG, Bonnier JJ. Modeling of (coronary) laser-angioplasty. Lasers in Surgery and Medicine 1985; 5: 219-234.

26. van Gemert MJC, Welch AJ, Bonnier JJM, Valvano JW, Yoon G, and Rastegar S. Some physical concepts in laser angioplasty. Seminars in Interventional Radiology 1986; 3: 27-38.

27. Geschwind RJ, Boussignac G, Teisseira B, et al. Conditions for effective Nd-YAG laser angioplasty. British Heart Journal 1984; 52: 484-489.

28. Gezondheidsraad. Hartchirurgie. The Hague, The Netherlands. 9 July 1984.

29. Ginsburg R, Kim DS, Cuthener D, Toth J, Mitchell RS. Salvage of an ischemic limb by laser angioplasty: description of a new technique. Clinical Cardiology 1984; 7: 54-58.

30. Ginsburg R, Wexler L, Mitchell RS, Proffit D. Percutaneous transluminal laser angioplasty for treatment of peripheral vascular disease, clinical experience with 16 patients. Radiology 1985; 156: 619-624.

31. Health Technology Assessment Reports, 1984. Assessment of carbon dioxide lasers in head and neck surgery. Washington, DC: National Center for Health Services Research.

32. Health Technology Assessment Reports, 1984. Assessment of Nd:YAG laser for posterior capsulotomies. Washington, DC: National Center for Health Services Research.

33. Health Technology Assessment Reports, 1984. Assessment of laser trabeculoplasty (LTP) for open angle glaucoma. Washington, DC: National Center for Health Services Research.

34. Isner Jm, Clarke RH. The current status of lasers in the treatment of cardiovascular disease. IEEE Journal of Quantum Electronics 1984; QE-20: 1406-1409.

35. Jacobs M. The light fantastic, lasers brighten the future. The Futurist, pp. 36-38, December 1985.

36. Kastler A. Birth of the maser and laser. Nature 1985; 316: 307-309.

37. Key MH. Laboratory production of X-ray lasers. Nature 1985; 316: 314-318.

38. Kiefhaber P, Nath G, Moritz K. Endoscopic control of massive gastrointestinal hemorrhage by irradiation with a high power neodymium YAG laser. Progress in Surgery 1977; 15: 140-155.

39. Lahaye CTW, van Gemert MJC. Optimal laser parameters for port wine stain therapy: a theoretical approach. Physics in Medicine and Biology 1985; 30: 573-587.

40. Laser report. Market supplement. Appendix to a Proposal submitted to the Texas Advanced Technology Program from the University of Texas at Austin. A.J. Welch and C.R. Denham, Principal Investigators, 1985.

41. Letokhov VS. Laser biology and medicine. Nature 1985; 316: 325-330.

42. Livesay JJ, Cooley DA. Laser coronary endarterectomy: proposed treatment for diffuse coronary atherosclerosis. Texas Heart Institute Journal 1984; 11: 276-279.

43. Livesay JJ, Johnnsen WE, Sutter LV, Klima T, Painvin A, Follette DM. Experimental technique of laser coronary endarterectomy and its immediate effects on atherosclerotic plaques in cadaver hearts. Texas Heart Institute Journal 1984; 11: 280-285.

44. Maddox J. Why celebrate laser birthday? Nature 1985; 316: 291.

45. Martin EC, Fankuchen EI, Karlson KB et al. Angioplasty for femoral artery occlusion: comparison with surgery. American Journal of Radiology 1981; 137: 915-919.

46. Mohr FW, Schoeneich G, Kirchhoff PG, Greulich O, Wolfrum J, Lenz W. Influence of excimer laser irradiation on human cardiovascular tissue. Lasers in Medical Science 1986; 1: 309.

47. Morelli JG, Tan OT, Garden J, Margolis R, Seki Y, Boll J, Carney JM, Angerson RR, Furumoto H, Parrish JA. Tunable dye laser (577 um) treatment of port wine stains. Lasers in Surgery and Medicine 1986; 6: 94-99.

48. Morse PH. Laser treatment for retinal vascular diseases. Annals of Ophthalmology 1985; 17: 156-162.

49. New laser role for diabetes eyed. Science News. 1985; 128: 377.

50. Office of Technology Assessment. The implications of cost-effectiveness analysis of medical technology. Washington, DC; US Government Printing Office, 1980.

51. Office of Technology Assessment. Policy implications of the computed tomography (CT) scanner. Washington, DC: US Government Printing Office, 1978.

52. Patel C.K.N. Lasers. In: Committee on Science, Engineering, and Public Policy, The Outlook for Science and Technology, the Next Five Years, Volume III. Washington, DC: National Academy Press, 1982, pp. 143-166.

53. Pratesi R. High-power semiconductor lasers in medicine. Lasers in Medical Science 1986; 1: 273 (abstract).

54. Quigley MR, Bailes JE, Kwaan HC, Cerullo LJ, Brown JT, Lastre C, Monma D. Microvascular anastomosis using the milliwatt CO_2 laser. Lasers in Surgery and Medicine 1985; 5: 357-365.

55. Rutgeerts P, Geboes K, Vantrappen G. Randomized comparision of contact and non-contact Nd-YAG laser therapy for rectal carcinoma. Lasers in Medical Science 1986; 1: 280 (abstract).

56. Sandeman DR. Photodynamic therapy in the managment of malignant gliomas: a review. Lasers in Medical Science 1986; 1: 163-174.

57. Sharp F, Jordan JA eds. Gynaecological laser surgery: proceedings of the fifteenth study group of the Royal College of Obstetricians and Gynaecologists. New York: Perinatology Press, 1986.

58. Shumaker BP, Lutz MD, Haas GP, Hetzel F. Practical clinical use of laser photodynamic therapy in the treatment of bladder carcinoma in situ. Lasers in Medical Science 1986; 1: 257-261.

59. Star WM. The state of the art of photodynamic therapy. Lasers in Medicine Science 1986; 1: 274 (abstract).

60. Stichting Informatie Centrum Gezondheidszorg - Ziekenfonden en Particuliere Verzekering. Het jaarboek 1984. Landelijke medische registratie. Utrecht.

61. Stuurgroep Toekomstscenario's Gezondheidszorg (STG). Het hart van de toekomst, de toekomst van het hart. Scenario's over hart en vaatziekten 1985-2010. The Hague, 1986.

62. Swain CP, Kirkham JS, Salmon PR, Bown SG, Northfield TC. Controlled trial of Nd-YAG laser photocoagulation in bleeding peptic ulcers. Lancet 1986; 1: 1113-1116.

63. Watson G, Wickham J. The use of a laser for fragmenting ureteric calculi. Draft Chapter for Book edited by Martin van Gemert and Tom Boon.

APPENDIX E ACKNOWLEDGEMENTS

Working Group on Laser Applications

The Working Group on Laser Applications met once, on 10 June 1986, to discuss a draft report on the technical aspects of lasers and proposed assumptions concerning future applications of lasers in coronary artery disease. The Working Group did not meet subsequently, but did review drafts of the report.

Dr. J.R.M. Bonnier
Catharina Ziekenhuis Eindhoven

Dr. C. Borst
Academisch Ziekenhuis Utrecht

Prof. dr. A.J. Dunning
Academisch Medisch Centrum Amsterdam

Dr. ir. M.J.C. van Gemert
St. Joseph Ziekenhuis Eindhoven

Dr. R. Naaborg
Nationale Raad voor de Volksgezondheid
Zoetermeer

Dr. E.G.M. Stassen
Reinier de Graaf Gasthuis Delft

Dr. W.J.M. Wils
Wils Systeem Analyse
's-Gravenhage

Other Contractors and Consultants

Dr. ir. M.J.C. van Gemert drafted parts of the report on lasers and reviewed the entire draft several times.

Dr. W.J.M. Wils did the computer work on the coronary artery disease model and the implications of lasers in the future.

The draft report was also reviewed, especially the parts dealing with economics, by Dr. Martin Buxton of Brunel University, England, and Dr. Frank de Charro of Erasmus University.

The total output of the project is as follows:

Volume 1	General Considerations and Policy Conclusions
Volume 2	Future Technological Changes
Volume 3	Developments in the Regeneration, Repair and Reorganization of Nervous Tissue
Volume 4	Health Care Applications of Lasers: The Future Treatment of Coronary Artery Disease
Volume 5	Developments in Genetic Testing
Volume 6	Applications of the New Biotechnology: The Case of Vaccines
Volume 7	Computer-Assisted Medical Imaging
Volume 8	Potentials for Home Care Technology

GPSR Compliance

The European Union's (EU) General Product Safety Regulation (GPSR) is a set of rules that requires consumer products to be safe and our obligations to ensure this.

If you have any concerns about our products, you can contact us on ProductSafety@springernature.com

In case Publisher is established outside the EU, the EU authorized representative is:

Springer Nature Customer Service Center GmbH
Europaplatz 3
69115 Heidelberg, Germany

Batch number: 10607330

Printed by Printforce, the Netherlands